W9-BTH-897

THE EAT FAT, GET THIN

COOKBOOK

ALSO BY MARK HYMAN, MD

———————

Eat Fat, Get Thin

The Blood Sugar Solution 10-Day Detox Diet Cookbook

The Blood Sugar Solution 10-Day Detox Diet

The Blood Sugar Solution Cookbook

The Blood Sugar Solution

The Daniel Plan

The Daniel Plan Cookbook

UltraPrevention

UltraMetabolism

The Five Forces of Wellness (CD)

The UltraMetabolism Cookbook

The UltraThyroid Solution

The UltraSimple Diet

The UltraMind Solution

Six Weeks to an UltraMind (CD)

UltraCalm (CD)

THE EAT FAT, GET THIN COOKBOOK

More Than 175 Delicious Recipes for Sustained Weight Loss and Vibrant Health

Mark Hyman, MD

Food photography by Leela Cyd

LITTLE, BROWN AND COMPANY

New York   Boston   London

This book is intended to supplement, not replace, the advice of a trained health professional. If you know or suspect that you have a health problem, you should consult a health professional. The author and publisher specifically disclaim any liability, loss, or risk, personal or otherwise, that is incurred as a consequence, directly or indirectly, of the use and application of any of the contents of this book.

Copyright © 2016 by Hyman Enterprises, LLC

Hachette Book Group supports the right to free expression and the value of copyright. The purpose of copyright is to encourage writers and artists to produce the creative works that enrich our culture.

The scanning, uploading, and distribution of this book without permission is a theft of the author's intellectual property. If you would like permission to use material from the book (other than for review purposes), please contact permissions@hbgusa.com. Thank you for your support of the author's rights.

Little, Brown and Company
Hachette Book Group
1290 Avenue of the Americas, New York, NY 10104
littlebrown.com

First Edition: November 2016

Little, Brown and Company is a division of Hachette Book Group, Inc. The Little, Brown name and logo are trademarks of Hachette Book Group, Inc.

The publisher is not responsible for websites (or their content) that are not owned by the publisher.

The Hachette Speakers Bureau provides a wide range of authors for speaking events. To find out more, go to hachettespeakersbureau.com or call (866) 376-6591.

Food stylist: Ayda Robana
Food photographer: Leela Cyd

Library of Congress Cataloging-in-Publication Data
Names: Hyman, Mark, author.
Title: The eat fat, get thin cookbook : more than 175 delicious recipes for sustained weight loss and vibrant health / Mark Hyman, MD.
Description: First edition. | New York: Little, Brown and Company, [2016] | Includes index.
Identifiers: LCCN 2016026941 | ISBN 978-0-316-31750-4
Subjects: LCSH: Reducing diets. | High-protein diet. | Reducing diets—Recipes. | LCGFT: Cookbooks.
Classification: LCC RM222.2 H96342 2016 | DDC 641.5/638—dc23 LC record available at https://lccn.loc.gov/2016026941

10 9 8 7 6 5 4 3 2 1

LSC-C

Printed in the United States of America

This book is dedicated to anyone who has suffered through a low-fat diet.
It's time to eat food that tastes good and is good for you.

Contents

Contents

THE EAT FAT, GET THIN

COOKBOOK

Introduction

"I had been overweight for many years, mostly from my unhealthy eating habits. *Eat Fat, Get Thin* appealed to me because the instructions were easy to follow.

"My results were miraculous. I have lost over 50 pounds. I was an insulin-dependent type 2 diabetic and was able to get off of diabetes and blood pressure medication on the fourth day. My A1C after two months on the program was 6.2, which was lower than during the 15-plus years on medication. My heartburn was gone on day one. My blood pressure has been well within normal range, sometimes lower. I no longer suffer from stiff and achy joints and have not felt this good since I can't remember when. I feel like I am in my 30s again, and I'm 68 years old. My family and friends cannot believe the huge transformation." —Joanne S.

I've seen thousands of patients just like Joanne—people who have tried countless diets and exercise plans, yet have been unable to achieve their health goals. That's because typical diets don't work.

I know that might sound crazy, but hear me out. Typical diets combine calorie deprivation with tasteless foods, which is a recipe for failure. It's simply too hard to keep cravings at bay when you feel deprived and aren't enjoying the food you do eat. Sugar addiction always seems to rear its ugly head, causing people to fall off the wagon. The problem with most diets is that they lack the key ingredient that actually makes food taste good and cuts your hunger: fat!

This is what makes the *Eat Fat, Get Thin* Plan different from other diets. It's not about deprivation or bland foods; it's about eating foods that nourish the whole body, while making your taste buds happy and fixing the hormones that make you hungry and gain weight.

Decades of brainwashing have left many of us afraid of one of the body's most necessary nutrients. I can't tell you how many patients I've had to coach, using baby steps, to eat coconut oil and avocados, or how many people have come to my house and been horrified to see me blending grass-fed butter into my coffee. I understand these responses, since I, too, had fat phobia at one point. I spent years eating a low-fat diet and recommending it to all my patients. The idea of promoting fat, especially saturated fat, in a healthy diet seemed outrageous.

It's not hard to understand where this fat fear came from. For years, doctors, scientists, the media, and even our government told us that eating fat causes weight gain and heart disease. These two myths, based on a few faulty studies, started a huge war on fat. Fats were soon replaced by carbs, sugar, and chemicals ("low fat" is usually code for "high sugar"), leading to one of the worst disease epidemics of all time. Type 2 diabetes in America has tripled since the 1980s, and researchers estimate that one in three Americans will have diabetes by 2050.

We now know that sugars and carbs, not fats, are the true causes of obesity and heart disease. Overconsumption of processed carbohydrates causes a spike in the body's production of the hormone insulin, which increases the storage of fat, especially dangerous belly fat. And that is just the start of the damage that sugar can do to your body.

Dietary fat, on the other hand, does not cause a spike in insulin. Unlike eating carbs, eating fat makes your body burn fat, rather than store it. Fats like butter and coconut oil, which were once maligned, are now being touted for their metabolism-boosting properties and the way they suppress hunger, lower triglycerides, reduce fat storage, and even improve athletic performance. Olive oil, or what I like to call liquid gold, has been shown to prevent heart disease, cancer, and diabetes. Healthy fats—such as avocados, wild fatty fish, nuts and seeds, and coconut and olive oils—also reduce inflammation in the body, help your brain perform better, and increase your overall energy. When you make healthy fats part of a low-glycemic (low sugar and starch), real- and whole-food diet, you can absolutely heal your body.

Digging through the research on fat over the last ten years has been life changing for me, in my practice and in my personal life. When I started to recommend fat to my own patients, I saw some of them lose one hundred or more pounds and even reverse type 2 diabetes. I had never witnessed such dramatic transformations before.

I began including more fats in my diet as well, and I noticed a shift in my own health. After getting off processed carbs and increasing my fat intake, not only did I have more mental focus and clarity, but I lost fifteen pounds and my love handles turned into a six-pack without my exercising any more than I had previously. I'm now eating more calories and losing more weight, and I eat fat with every single meal! For breakfast I'll often have an omelet or a frittata cooked in grass-fed butter or a smoothie made with nuts and seeds, coconut milk, and/or an avocado. For lunch I might have a big salad with wild fatty fish like salmon or sardines, plus avocados and pumpkin seeds with plenty of extra-virgin olive oil, and for dinner, grass-fed lamb (keeping the fat on it, of course) paired with different veggies and more olive oil on top. The satisfaction of eating increases dramatically when you cook your food with real, healthy fats. Fat is what makes food taste good.

With the help of my friend Chef Frank Giglio, I've put together more than 175 deeply satisfying and delicious recipes to share with you. You can use these recipes before, during, and after your twenty-one-day *Eat Fat, Get Thin* Plan, which you can find in my book *Eat Fat, Get Thin* and in Part II of this book. I've also included recipes that are specifically designed to be used after the twenty-one-day plan. They fall into what I like to call the Pegan Diet. The Pegan Diet, which I explain in Chapter 4, combines the best of the Paleo and vegan diets. It is the way that I eat 90 percent of the time, and I've never felt better. I'm sharing the recipes in this book because I want everyone to feel this way—satisfied, satiated, and full of energy and vitality.

Let's take back our kitchens and take back our health. It all starts in these pages.

PART I

THE BASICS

So many of you have already experienced monumental changes in your health. Some of you may just be getting started, and others might be looking for a reset to get back on track. Wherever you are on this journey, I hope this cookbook serves as inspiration to continue to seek the best version of yourself. In these next chapters, I'll give you my best tips for creating a safe and joyful space for healing and thriving, and we'll recap the *Eat Fat, Get Thin* Plan, so that you feel fully prepared to enthusiastically and easily take control of your health.

1

Seven Big Ideas

Before we get started with the *Eat Fat, Get Thin* Plan, I want to take you through some key principles that have helped me and my patients on the journey to optimal health. You might be familiar with some of these concepts, and in that case, consider them helpful reminders. Some are related to food, others are more about emotional health, but all are necessary on the path toward vibrant well-being. I call them the Seven Big Ideas.

BIG IDEA 1: FOOD IS NOT LIKE MEDICINE — IT *IS* MEDICINE

Nothing beats the true healing power of real food. Normally, by the time patients come to a Functional Medicine doctor like me, they've exhausted what conventional medicine offers. Conventional medicine is by far the best for acute illness. But food is the best medicine for chronic disease. It works faster and better, and is cheaper than medication. And all the side effects are good ones. Remember Joanne's story—off insulin, diabetes medication, and blood-pressure medication in four days after fifteen years of struggling. No drug can do what (real) food can do.

Nutrigenomics is the idea that food is information and that that information is always communicating with our genes, turning on messages that foster health and/or disease. If every part of each food we eat contains valuable information for our bodies that affects gene expression, then why, for so long, were we obsessed with focusing only on one tiny part of the food we consume: the number of calories? Calories matter, but far less than the information or instructions in food that control our genes, hormones, immune system, enzymes, and even our gut flora or microbiome with every single bite.

Imagine what message you're sending your body when you eat nutritionally empty foods such as cheeseburgers, potato chips, French fries, and cupcakes. Compare this to the message sent by plant foods, which are packed with powerful antioxidants and phytochemicals that your body needs. Unfortunately, there are some foods, like fat, that continue to be demonized even though they send important and very powerful messages to our cells.

A decade ago, when I started to really dig into the research on dietary fats, I found undeniably clear evidence that in the absence of refined sugars and processed carbohydrates, healthy fats shut down cravings, speed up metabolism, and can help prevent and reverse heart disease, *not* cause it. But because we were (and still are) a country focused on calories, and because fats contain more calories than processed carbohydrates or sugars, many "experts" continued to dismiss this macronutrient because it is more "calorie dense." I'm happy to report that several recent studies have shown how incredibly powerful and healing good fats are and that saturated fat is *not* the villain it was made out to be for so long. And that fat actually helps you lose weight, not gain weight. We need to put dangerous low-fat diets behind us as we embrace the fact that we have the most healing treatments in the world available right at our fingertips, and they come from the "farmacy," not the pharmacy.

BIG IDEA 2: FOOD AND FAT ARE *NOT* THE ENEMY

Our relationship with food is one of the most important relationships in our lives. It's also one of our first relationships. From day one, food nourishes us and enables us to live and thrive. But like any long-term relationship, this one can become toxic. Sadly, fear around food and fat is more prevalent than ever. We have been convinced that fat makes us fat and that all calories are equal and should be counted as such. But metabolism is not a math problem. It is about the quality and composition of our food and the hormones and molecules they influence.

Before you start the twenty-one-day plan, I want you to take out your journal or a piece of paper and really think about your relationship with food and fat. Ask yourself the following questions:

- What beliefs am I holding on to about fat?
- What is my relationship to or belief about a fat-free diet?
- How have low-fat diets worked for me in the past? What happened when I tried them?
- What worries or fears do I have about including fat in my diet?

Answering these questions is the first step in letting go of any negative relationship with food and fat. If you are a chronic dieter, the *Eat Fat, Get Thin* Plan is perfect for you. Once you clear out the junk and reset your body, you can move on to a way of eating that allows room for pleasure foods while focusing on eating real, whole foods most of the time. You'll be able to think of food as a friend who nourishes you and brings you joy instead of an enemy you have to fear or battle every day.

BIG IDEA 3: BE YOUR OWN DOCTOR

Conventional medicine focuses on naming diseases based on specific body location instead of underlying cause. Doctors say you have liver, kidney, brain, or heart disease, but this approach tells you nothing about the *cause*.

Instead of asking what disease you have and what drug should be used to treat it, we must ask what underlying causes led to the disease or illness. I empower my patients to do a little bit of investigative work, specific to them, because no two bodies are the same. One person's weight gain might be the result of mercury toxicity, while another's stems from imbalances in gut flora that have led to irritable bowel syndrome. Become a detective.

What works for your neighbor might not work for you. Some people do better with a higher-fat diet and others do better with more carbs such as sweet potatoes or small amounts of whole grains (no one does well on lots of processed carbs or flours). Experiment with these foods, and while you experiment, keep track of your findings in a food journal, taking note of how you feel after your meals. Your body will give you clues each day. Inquisitiveness and intuition will help you discover where your ailments are coming from and what might help treat them. We just have to listen and pay attention.

BIG IDEA 4: WEIGHT LOSS — EVERYONE IS DIFFERENT

Eat Fat, Get Thin is more than a catchy title — it's the truth. Dietary fat can actually speed up your metabolism and help you lose weight. Even better, once you start this program, you'll find that it's a gateway to something much bigger than the numbers on the scale.

Weight loss happens differently for everyone. You might find that you lose more weight in the beginning of the program or at the end, or it might happen steadily all the way through. We're all different and have different paces and needs. Be patient with your body. Make sure you're drinking enough water and moving your bowels every day. Get at least thirty minutes of exercise a day (ideally including high-intensity interval training) to speed up your metabolism and to get the endorphins flowing; they lift your mood and make challenges seem less daunting. Endorphins make you feel good, and when you feel good, you tend to make healthier choices for your body. Also, recognize that weight loss might take some time. Three weeks can create a huge shift in your body, but it's still just three weeks. Depending on how many years of poor eating, lack of exercise, or other issues have preceded the program, we may have to dig deeper. Environmental toxins, nutritional imbalances, hormonal imbalances, a damaged gut, and stress can all contribute to unexplained weight gain. A program like *Eat Fat, Get Thin* is a great starting point, but if you suspect that there is a deeper issue, or if you're struggling along the way, I recommend seeking the help of a Functional Medicine practitioner (www.functionalmedicine.org).

BIG IDEA 5: ASK WHY

Learn more, love more, be a better doctor, be a better father, reach more people, heal the planet, end obesity. These are just some of my personal goals, and my desire to achieve these goals is what motivates me to put my health first. Anytime I feel stressed and fail to adequately take care of myself, I always stop and remember why. Why is my health important? My health is important because I can't show up as the best version of myself and go after my goals if I feel sick, unhealthy, unbalanced, or stressed.

Before you start this program, and as you go through it, I want you to ask yourself *why* you're doing it. Maybe you want to increase your energy so that you can keep up with your kids or grandkids, or perhaps you want more mental clarity to perform better at work or school. Maybe you want to feel good in your own skin so you can have better relationships with the people you love. Whatever they are, it's essential to remind yourself of your own personal goals on a daily basis. Not only are they more achievable when you feel energized, but you get to enjoy the journey as you work toward them, which is just as, if not more, important.

The first step is really clearly setting your goals. Ask yourself what's important to you and how you can live in ways that are in alignment with this vision. I have never met anyone who wakes up in the morning and says, "It's my goal to get fatter and sicker and create disease." So, odds are this is not your goal; therefore, why would you make choices that lead to this outcome? Chances are, you want the complete opposite for yourself. You want to feel good, look good, and cook delicious and healthy meals that make you feel satisfied. You want to prepare this food and share these benefits with the people in your life as well, so how can you make decisions that support this outcome? You want to design your life to create health and well-being, not disease or "feeling like crap." Think about how you can redesign your life to make healthy choices automatic.

Just sticking with the recommendations of this plan is not always enough to keep the motivation going, but taking a look at your goals and reminding yourself of the bigger picture will help you to keep your perspective.

BIG IDEA 6: FRIEND-POWER, NOT WILLPOWER

In 2014, I wrote *The Daniel Plan* with my friends Pastor Rick Warren and Dr. Daniel Amen. We took Pastor Warren's congregations through a six-week challenge based on the principles of Functional Medicine to change biology and optimize health and the power of social connections and positive peer pressure to change behavior. We used the power of social networks to hold people accountable and help them reach their health goals.

The results were astounding. The congregations lost a quarter of a million pounds in ten months. They also improved things like depression, autoimmune disease, diabetes, high blood pressure, and acne. One day, Pastor Warren said, "Every *body* needs a buddy. Getting healthy is a team sport." Those words stuck with me. The reason we experienced such profound results during our first trial of The Daniel Plan was because the congregation was playing as a team.

Instead of using willpower, I recommend using friend-power. If you can do this program with a family member or friend, that's awesome! You can also start a community meet-up for intentional eaters in your area, find a coach, or join our online community (www.drhyman.com /community). You may be surprised at how many people have been wanting to change their habits but were waiting for someone else to encourage them. Creating a community of like-minded people will always lead to a more favorable outcome for everybody, as group encouragement goes a long way. Humans are pack animals and social creatures; we're meant to rely on one another for support.

Granted, you may occasionally run into a naysayer who feels threatened by the lifestyle changes you're making. I call these "food pushers." Just have that one piece of cake—*what's the big deal?* they say. I find that people who react negatively to my eating habits often behave that way because they are questioning their own diet and lifestyle. It can be hard, but try to take the high road. Stick to what feels good, trust that you are making the best decisions for yourself, and don't pay any attention to what the haters say. In fact, as you're making changes, now might be a good time to (gently) cut the negative energy loose.

BIG IDEA 7: LEAVE THE JUDGMENT BEHIND

I recently came across this quote: "If you had a friend who talked to you the way that you talked to yourself, you would have ditched that friend a long time ago." How true is that? We are our own harshest critics. So I challenge you to now become your own best friend. Instead of looking in the mirror and judging yourself for everything you believe to be wrong with your body, why not praise yourself for taking this huge step toward better health?

Your body is listening to everything you say. Indulging in self-deprecation leads to stress; stress wreaks havoc on your health. And if you find yourself making a bad decision or going off course during this journey, leave the guilt behind, too. It's just as toxic, and it doesn't help you at all. Be like your car's GPS: when you veer off course, gently remind yourself to make a U-turn. The diet and exercise industry is filled with borderline harmful messages like "no pain, no gain," and we have been taught that looking good has to feel bad. Killing ourselves at the gym, forcing ourselves to eat foods we find unenjoyable, or, even worse, starving and denying ourselves is a recipe for disaster.

I encourage you, instead, to find joy in this process. Joy makes food taste better. Every single recipe in this book has been created and taste tested for maximum pleasure and flavor. I am not an advocate of suffering to become the best version of yourself. The best version of yourself is healthy *and* happy. The best version of yourself loves to be active, play in the sunshine, and create beautiful, wholesome meals. This collection of recipes is designed to nourish that best version of you, with recipes that make your mouth water *and* make you feel good.

Everyone's path is different, but we are all in this together. If you are reading this book, you are interested in bettering yourself, and that's incredibly exciting. Know that the road to your own personal vibrant health can absolutely be enjoyable.

Now that we've prepared our minds, it is time to prepare our kitchens!

Be sure to talk with your health care provider before embarking on this journey, especially if you're on any medications or dealing with chronic illness.

2

Getting Started: The *Eat Fat, Get Thin* Plan

In the recent documentary series *Cooked*, my friend Michael Pollan discussed the correlation between time spent in the kitchen and obesity rates. No surprise here: As the average amount of time that we spend in the kitchen has gone down, obesity rates have gone up. I understand where the desire to outsource cooking comes from; my schedule is pretty jam-packed, and some days even the thought of walking into the kitchen can be daunting. But what is the cost of choosing convenience over real nourishment? A sick nation. A world in which families are disconnected and spending more time in front of their TVs or hunched over a screen, mindlessly eating processed takeout, and less time with one another eating real food. And the truth is that simple cooking doesn't take a long time, and it is not inconvenient or expensive. It is a bunch of propaganda the food industry has convinced us is true. Anyway, how convenient or cheap is it to be sick and fat and tired and have chronic diseases and take medication your entire life? Not so much!

The only way to ensure that you and your family are eating safe, nutritious food is to get back into the kitchen and make the time to connect with what you're eating. You should be able to identify every single ingredient in your meals and snacks. Think about how long it took for that ingredient to get from the farm to your fork. If it made a pit stop at a factory, or if it was made in a factory, and sometimes even if it sat on a truck for days traveling across the country to get to you, it may not be good enough for your body. Remember, you deserve real food. It's a birthright of being human.

The first step to reconnecting with your kitchen is to make it a safe zone by filling it with foods that nourish and removing foods that harm. This will ensure that you automatically make the right choices, especially if you're pressed for time and looking for something quick. The same goes for your backpack, purse, car, school locker, and so on; anywhere you look for food, you should have only the good stuff available. Think of all the willpower it takes to have to battle cravings for junk food that's right under your nose, and all the other places that energy could go instead! Set yourself up for success by making your home and environment a safe zone free of foods that harm you and make you feel bad, and full of foods that heal and make you feel good.

The first part of the *Eat Fat, Get Thin* Plan is the preparation stage, which I recommend starting two days before your program. This involves giving your kitchen a makeover so that you can prepare these flavorful meals quickly and easily and complete your twenty-one-day *Eat Fat, Get Thin* Plan with success. Even if you're using this book just for recipes, I still recommend detoxifying your kitchen, as it makes it so much easier to choose healthy options.

Next, I'll cover everything that you'll eat and drink during the twenty-one-day plan, and finally, I'll lay out the Pegan Diet, which is the diet that you'll transition to after the twenty-one-day plan.

Thousands of people have participated in the *Eat Fat, Get Thin* Plan, and they've experienced significant weight loss, a decrease in cravings, and balanced blood sugar and blood pressure, as well as a *huge* reduction in symptoms of many different diseases and health issues. That is how powerful this program is, and it all starts with the food that we eat. The benefits come from using food as medicine to create health. The pounds and symptoms drop off as side effects.

So let's get started with your kitchen makeover. Have your trash bag and recycling bin ready to completely remove all of the following items from your cupboards and fridge:

- Anything containing hydrogenated oils or refined vegetable oils (like corn or soybean). These oils are highly unstable and inflammatory. We were told that vegetable oils were healthy alternatives to butter and lard, but they actually contribute to heart disease, diabetes, cancer, and a number of other ailments. Get rid of them. Bonus: Getting rid of these ingredients means you pretty much eliminate all packaged and processed foods, since most of them contain these oils. So you're eliminating excess sugar and salt in one fell swoop! The average salad dressing is made from soybean oil and high-fructose corn syrup. What a way to ruin your vegetables!

- All fake foods. Get rid of anything that's processed or contains preservatives, additives, or dyes. Get rid of anything labeled "fat free" or "low fat" or "natural flavors," which are not really natural at all. Those words almost always mean that sugar or additives have taken the place of healthy fat.

- Anything containing artificial sweeteners (Splenda, sorbitol, aspartame, etc.) or processed sugar, especially high-fructose corn syrup.

- All processed meats, such as deli meats. The World Health Organization has singled these out as major causes of disease, including cancer.

While the above items are toxic and should be avoided completely, you might be able to incorporate some of the following foods back into your diet after the twenty-one-day plan. But you'll want to keep them out of sight for three weeks:

- Any product containing gluten. An undiagnosed gluten intolerance can cause a whole host of problems, including autoimmune conditions, leaky gut, dementia, and diabetes. Most of us generally feel better when we avoid it, especially in the highly processed and often chemical- and GMO-filled gluten products in this country. And the main form we consume gluten in is flour, which is worse than table sugar and is highly addictive.

- Non-gluten grains. These include rice, quinoa, barley, millet, or any other grains. Whole grains can be a wonderful part of a healthy diet, but they are still starch and can spike blood sugar and insulin. They also create gut problems and inflammation for some people, so we avoid them during the first twenty-one days of the program.

- All dairy products. Dairy is often full of hormones and antibiotics. The only dairy I recommend is grass-fed butter or ghee, and some people do okay with raw cheese, yogurt, or milk from pastured animals, but save those personal experiments until after the twenty-one days. Ideally, use ghee—which removes the casein and whey (the allergenic proteins in dairy).

- Beans. They contain a fair amount of starch, and for blood sugar issues, they aren't ideal. They can also cause digestive problems, something we're trying to avoid on the program.

- All fruit, with the exception of berries, pomegranate seeds, watermelon, lemons, limes, and kiwi. Fruit is full of antioxidants, beneficial fiber, and nutrients, but I have seen plenty of patients overindulge in fruits as a substitute for their sugary snacks. When you're trying to lose weight or balance your blood sugar, it's best to stick with a small amount of low-glycemic fruit. A good rule of thumb is to eat primarily fruit that's local and in season, which drastically limits the amount of fruit we eat for most of the year. Remember, the natural packaging that fruit comes in has a purpose, as nature always knows what it's doing! When you do eat fruit, try to eat the pith and the skin, too, as the added fiber slows down blood sugar and the bitterness of the pith aids in digestion.

- All alcohol. Regular alcohol consumption can cause inflammation, which can lead to weight gain, pre-diabetes, and diabetes. It also creates strong and often uncontrollable cravings and can put a large strain on your gut and liver health. Use in moderation (three to five drinks per week at most) once you're done with the program, but avoid alcohol for these three weeks.

FILL YOUR FRIDGES AND STOCK YOUR PANTRIES

Now that you've removed the poison from your pantries (or the foods that can sabotage your health), we can talk about all of the delicious foods you'll get to eat every day. When creating a healthy meal or snack, there are three types of foods to focus on. It's more about all the good, delicious things you can eat rather than the things you can't.

- First: slow carbs or nonstarchy plant foods. These include green leafy veggies, broccoli, mushrooms, tomatoes, peppers, bok choy, and many, many more. When it comes to slow carbs, the options are endless. These foods should make up 75 percent of your plate. I place an emphasis on nonstarchy veggies because they contain potent antioxidants, vitamins, and minerals that have powerful healing properties and are low in sugar or starch. On the *Eat Fat, Get Thin* Plan you can occasionally include starchy veggies (beets, parsnips, sweet potatoes, and yams) for dinner.
- Second: protein. On average, you should be getting four to six ounces of protein with each meal. This is about the size of the palm of your hand. Protein is necessary for appetite control and muscle synthesis. Muscle is your metabolic engine. Your protein sources will come from pasture-raised eggs, nuts and seeds, grass-fed and organic meats, clean fish, and non-GMO whole soy foods.
- Last but certainly not least: fats. The right fats can improve your mood, skin, hair, and nails, while protecting you against type 2 diabetes, dementia, cancer, and much more. Healthy fats are the best source of energy for your body and keep your metabolism and fat-burning mechanism running as they're meant to. And they are the key to cutting cravings and curbing your appetite. Be sure to eat at least four to five servings of fat per day. Healthy fats can be found in foods like wild fatty fish (sardines, mackerel, herring, wild salmon), grass-fed meat or organic poultry (skin and fat left on), nuts and seeds, avocados, extra-virgin olive oil, and coconut oil.

Here are some examples of a fat serving:

- Extra-virgin coconut oil (1 tablespoon)
- Extra-virgin olive oil, avocado oil, macadamia oil, walnut oil, almond oil (1 tablespoon)
- MCT oil (1 to 2 tablespoons a day)
- Organic coconut milk (¼ cup)
- Avocado (½ to 1 avocado)
- Fatty fish like sardines, mackerel, herring, black cod, and wild salmon (4 to 6 ounces); aim to include these three to four times per week
- Nuts and seeds (2 to 3 handfuls)
- Olives (¼ cup)
- Grass-fed butter, clarified butter, or ghee (1 tablespoon); if you are allergic to dairy, just use ghee

The following is a cheat sheet listing all the approved foods and fats and the off-limits ones. You can photocopy these pages and keep them in your purse or wallet, or take a picture with your smartphone, and use them for easy reference when you're at the market.

Going Organic

When possible, choose organic, seasonal, and local produce. To help you prioritize when choices are limited, consult the Environmental Working Group's "Dirty Dozen" and "Clean Fifteen" lists, showing the foods you should always source organic due to pesticide use and/or skin thickness, and those you can safely buy when organic isn't an option. The expanded "Dirty Dozen" list includes apples, celery, sweet bell peppers, peaches, strawberries, nectarines, grapes, spinach, lettuce, cucumbers, blueberries, potatoes, grapes, kale, and all other green leafy veggies. Don't forget about the freezer section; you can often find organic fruits and vegetables there. Check out www.ewg.org for an updated list.

What to Eat		
	Focus on These Items…	*Avoid These Items…*
Fat (aim for 4 to 5 servings a day, all organic)	Nuts (except for peanuts), seeds, and nut butters: chia, flax, sesame, black sesame, sunflower, hemp seeds, pumpkin seeds, hazelnuts, macadamia nuts, pecans, walnuts, almonds, cashews Nut and seed milks: almond, Brazil nut, cashew, coconut, hemp Avocados, olives Ghee, grass-fed butter, coconut butter Oils (extra-virgin and cold-pressed): avocado, coconut, macadamia nut, MCT, olive, walnut, sesame	Dairy products (except for grass-fed butter and ghee; those are okay) (for 21 days) All refined vegetable oils: canola, corn, safflower, soy, sunflower (for the long term)
Animal foods/ protein (aim for 4 to 6 ounces of protein per meal, all grass-fed and organic). Can also be vegetable protein in form of non-GMO whole soy.	Bison, beef, elk, lamb, ostrich, venison Eggs, chicken, duck, turkey Lard, tallow, duck and goose fat (free-range, pasture-raised) Fresh or canned fatty fish: black cod, herring, mackerel, perch, sardines, scallops, wild salmon, anchovies Shellfish: clams, crab, mussels, oysters, scallops, shrimp Non-GMO tofu, tempeh	Legumes, beans (for 21 days) Processed meats: bacon, canned meats, hot dogs, salami (for the long term) High-mercury fish: king mackerel, tuna, swordfish, Chilean sea bass, halibut, lobster, marlin, shark, tilefish, orange roughy (for the long term). See www.nrdc.org for a guide to low-mercury fish.
Carbohydrates (raw, steamed, roasted, or sautéed; approximately 50 to 75 percent of your plate should be made up of nonstarchy veggies)	Artichokes, arugula, asparagus, avocados, bean sprouts (not alfalfa sprouts, which contain natural carcinogens), beet greens, bell peppers, broccoli, Brussels sprouts, cabbage, carrots (no juicing because it turns them into pure sugar), cauliflower, celery, chives, collard greens, dandelion greens, eggplant, endive, fennel, fresh herbs, garlic, ginger, green beans, hearts of palm, jalapeños, kale, lettuce,	Gluten, all grains (for 21 days) All fruit (with the exception of berries, kiwi, lemon, lime, pomegranate seeds, watermelon: ½ to 1 cup per day) (for 21 days)

	Focus on These Items…	Avoid These Items…
Carbohydrates *(continued)*	mushrooms, mustard greens, onions, radicchio, radishes, seaweeds (kelp, aramae, wakame, etc.), shallots, snap peas, snow peas, spinach, summer squash, Swiss chard, tomatoes, turnip greens, watercress, zucchini ½ to 1 cup of starchy veggies up to 4 times a week at dinner: beets, celeriac, parsnips, pumpkin, sweet potatoes, winter squash (butternut, kabocha, acorn, etc.)	
Drinks	Hot lemon water, sparkling water with lemon or lime, herbal or green teas, Bulletproof Coffee or Tea, bone broth	Alcohol (for 21 days) Soda, diet soda, milk, fruit juices, sports drinks (for the long term)
Other (condiments, spices, staples)	Almond flour, apple cider vinegar, arrowroot, balsamic vinegar, black peppercorn, coconut flour, coconut aminos, Dijon mustard, kelp noodles, kimchi, miso, nutritional yeast, organic vegetable and chicken stock, sea salt, spirulina, tahini, ume plum vinegar, unsweetened vanilla and chocolate (cacao) powder, wheat-free tamari, dried or fresh herbs and spices such as basil, cayenne pepper, chili powder, cinnamon, coriander, cardamom, ginger, cumin, onion powder, oregano, paprika, parsley, rosemary, sage, thyme, turmeric	Natural sweeteners: honey, maple syrup, raw sugar, etc. (for 21 days) Additives, preservatives, dyes, MSG (for the long term) Artificial sweeteners: Splenda, Equal, aspartame, sorbitol, xylitol, stevia (for the long term)

Some of the items listed in the approved section might be unfamiliar, but I promise that experimenting with them is well worth it. For example, we've included a recipe for pancakes (page 82) that uses coconut flour instead of regular flour. Trust me, you don't want to miss out on these pancakes! New and different ingredients help spice up your cooking routine so you're not stuck with the same few meals day after day. Let me introduce you to some of the new ingredients you will experiment with.

Almond Flour and Almond Meal

An alternative to grain-based flours, almond flour is made by blanching and grinding almonds into a fine powder. Almond meal is typically a coarser grind made with the skin still left on. Both can be used to bake breads, desserts, and crusts. They are full of protein and good fats, as well as vitamins and minerals.

Apple Cider Vinegar

I use apple cider vinegar in my salad dressings, sauces, and dips. It is anti-bacterial and antiviral, it helps combat constipation, and it can make your skin glow when taken daily.

Arrowroot

Arrowroot is a thickener that can be used in soups, stews, baked goods, and more. It is a great alternative to conventional thickeners like cornstarch.

Bone Broth

Bone broth contains powerful gut-healing properties. Chicken, beef, lamb, bison, venison, turkey, and/or duck bones are simmered for long periods of time with veggies and filtered water to create an immunity-supporting beverage that can be sipped on its own or added to other meals, soups, and stews. Great for kids, pets, and anyone with compromised digestion. You can get the recipe on page 128.

Bulletproof Coffee

Coffee is not a requirement on this program, but if you do enjoy coffee, Bulletproof Coffee, invented by my friend Dave Asprey, will change your life with its frothy goodness. Adding fat to your coffee can stop cravings and improve brain function and focus. To Bulletproof your beverage, blend 1 cup of coffee, 1 tablespoon of grass-fed butter or ghee, 1 tablespoon of coconut or MCT oil, and, if you like, ½ teaspoon of cinnamon and/or cocoa powder (for a mocha). If you aren't a coffee fan, you can also add fat to your tea using the same recipe. If you want to be dairy free you can use 1 tablespoon of organic cashew butter, which makes it creamy and delicious.

Chia Seeds

Chia seeds pack an antioxidant punch and are filled with omega-3 fatty acids and fiber to help feed friendly gut bacteria. They can be added to your smoothies, and since they absorb water easily, you can also use them to create puddings. We have a yummy recipe for chia seed pudding on page 87.

Coconut Aminos

Coconut aminos are a terrific alternative to soy sauce. They are made from coconut sap and have a similar consistency and taste to soy sauce, but they are gluten-free. They also contain minerals as well as vitamins B and C and can be used in stir-fries, soups, dips, and more. You can find them in your local health-food store or online.

Coconut Butter

Coconut butter is made from the meat of coconuts, and it has a thick, buttery consistency that I love using in my smoothies as a thickener. I also spread it on homemade, grain-free breads for a super-satiating snack. You can find it in the nut-butter section of most grocery stores or online.

Coconut Cream

An amazing whipped cream alternative! Coconut cream has a higher fat content than coconut milk, so you can whip it into a rich texture to top ice creams or add to your coffee drinks. A Bulletproof Coffee drink with whipped coconut cream is the most amazing (and healthy) treat! My favorite brand is Native Forest, which you can purchase online or at your local health-food store.

Coconut Flour

Just like almond flour, coconut flour makes a great substitute for grain-based flours. Coconut flour is made from dried coconut meat, and it's a bit sweeter than almond flour, so it's great for sweet breads and pancakes. It's an excellent source of fiber and helps balance blood sugar and eliminate cravings.

Flaxseeds

Flaxseeds are an ideal source of essential omega-3 fats, dietary fiber, and key vitamins and minerals. I like adding them to my smoothies and salads. They also help to combat constipation and keep blood sugar levels in check. Keep them refrigerated, especially if they are ground.

Ghee

Also known as clarified butter, ghee is made by melting butter, then simmering it over low heat until most of the water evaporates and the milk solids float to the top to be clarified off, leaving beneficial fat. In Ayurvedic medicine, ghee is used for its powerful healing properties. It's perfect for higher-temperature cooking since it stays stable at high heats. You can find a recipe for ghee on page 279.

Grass-fed Butter

The only other dairy product I recommend is grass-fed butter. Beef from cows that are fed only grain produces a much higher omega-6 content in comparison to grass-fed cows, and since omega-6 fats are more inflammatory, I suggest sticking to grass-fed butter. It's great for satiation, energy, and improved mood and brain function.

Hemp Seeds

Hemp seeds are gaining in popularity and with good reason, as they are a true powerhouse of nutritional benefit. They are a fantastic source of protein, iron, and magnesium. You can sprinkle them onto your salads or add them to your smoothies and baked goods.

Kelp Noodles

Ditch the pasta for good! Kelp noodles are a nutritionally dense alternative to grains, made from kelp, a kind of seaweed. They're really mineral-rich, so you can enjoy them without guilt. We've included a couple of kelp noodle recipes for you to try out.

Kimchi

Fermented foods have been rising in popularity over the years as gut health has taken center stage. Kimchi is a traditional Korean food that involves fermenting a variety of vegetables with probiotics. The result is a fiber- and nutrient-rich dish that can be cooked with other ingredients or served raw as a side (for the most gut benefit).

MCT Oil

MCT stands for medium-chain triglycerides, a fatty acid derived from coconut oil. Consider MCT oil a superfuel for your cells because it boosts fat burning and increases mental clarity. You can use it in your coffee and add it to smoothies, salads, or any other meal. You can find MCT oil on our resources page at www.eatfatgetthin.com/resources.

Miso

Fermenting soybeans creates this immunity-boosting superfood that can be used to make soups, sauces, and dressings. There are many different kinds of miso. Look for the ones that are fermented without grains.

Nutritional Yeast

Believe it or not, cheesy, creamy salads and sauces can be achieved without using dairy. Nutritional yeast is deactivated yeast that you can sprinkle onto your meals. It's one of my favorite condiments because it adds a delicious flavor and a cheesy texture, and it's a great source of energy-providing vitamin B_{12}.

Spirulina

A blue-green algae that's a wonderful source of B vitamins, protein, and iron, spirulina is another powerhouse food that can be eaten by meat eaters and vegetarians alike. Listing all of the benefits of spirulina would take up a whole page—let's just say I highly recommend it. I personally love to add it to smoothies and on top of salads, and a tiny bit goes a long way.

Tahini

Made from ground sesame seeds, and high in protein and healthy fat, tahini (alone or blended with other ingredients) makes the perfect dressing or dip for your vegetables. It's a great alternative to nut butters, especially for those who are allergic to nuts.

Teff Flour

Teff flour is a gluten-free flour made from a grain called teff and is traditionally used in Ethiopian cuisine to make bread. Teff is rich in protein, calcium, and iron. We've included a delicious bread made from teff in the recipes (page 253). You can find teff flour in health-food stores and online.

Tempeh

Made from fermented soybeans, tempeh has a dense texture with a good amount of protein, so if you're vegetarian or looking to experiment with a new food, try replacing the animal protein in recipes with tempeh. Fermented tempeh is a healthier alternative to processed soy products like tofu and TVP (textured vegetable protein).

Ume Plum Vinegar

Ume plum vinegar is made from fermented umeboshi plums. It has a unique salty-sour taste and can be used as a general seasoning or in soups, stocks, sauces, and stir-fries. It's also traditionally used as a detoxification aid and palate cleanser.

Wheat- and Gluten-Free Tamari

Instead of using soy sauce, try wheat-free tamari. It has a similar taste and is a significantly healthier, gluten-free option.

STOCK YOUR TOOLBOX

Experimenting with all of these delicious foods is much easier and a lot more fun when you have the right tools. Think of these tools as an investment in your health. Once I equipped myself with a great set of knives, a powerful blender, wooden cutting boards, and other quality kitchen essentials, I was much more excited about playing in the kitchen. The following tools are essential:

Blender (If you can invest in one, I would get a VitaMix. It will last a lifetime.)

Good set of knives (keep them sharp)

2 wooden cutting boards (one for animal foods, one for fruits and vegetables, and some people like to keep a third for onions and garlic)

Nonstick sauté pan, cast-iron pan, or both

8-quart stockpot

2-quart and 4-quart saucepans with lids

Several rimmed baking sheets

Several square and/or rectangular baking dishes

Food processor (sometimes a blender can be used instead, but a food processor is a handy kitchen tool to have as well)

Instant-read thermometer

Spatulas (metal and rubber)

Can opener

Colander

Measuring cups, metal for dry ingredients and glass for liquids

Measuring spoons

Mixing bowls

Wooden spoons

The following tools make cooking a little easier, but they are optional. You definitely don't have to go out and spend a ton of money and overhaul your kitchen to make this program work for you.

11-inch square nonstick stove-top griddle
Dutch oven
Grill pan
Steamer
Coffee grinder for flaxseeds and spices
Vegetable-steaming rack or basket
Citrus reamer
Rubber spatulas
Wire whisks
Spring tongs
Pliers or tweezers (for deboning fish)
Microplane graters/zesters in assorted sizes
Food mill
Natural parchment paper and foil
Cloth kitchen towels
Spirulizer (for making vegetable noodles)
Mandolin slicer
Vegetable peeler
Timer (most everyone's phone has one now)
Sealable glass containers in various sizes for storing food (preferred
    to plastic storage containers, as they don't leach plastic into
    your food)

STOCK YOUR MEDICINE CABINETS

Eating real, whole foods, and especially plant foods, is the most important part of your transformation toward optimal health. In the long run, plant foods are the best source of vitamins, minerals, phytonutrients, antioxidants, and fiber, but because of depleted soils, the vegetables and fruits we eat have fewer nutrients than plants grown in healthy organic soils.

Foundational support through supplementation is key to healing your gut, reducing inflammation, balancing blood sugar, and recovering from nutritional deficiencies. Here's a rundown of all the supplements you will need for your twenty-one-day plan (and they can be taken over the long term as well to maintain your health). You can purchase these as a full pack for ease and convenience at www.eatfatgetthin.com/resources, or purchase them individually at your local health-food store.

Supplement	Benefits	Daily Dosage
High-quality multivitamin and multimineral	*Contains all the B vitamins, antioxidants, and minerals you need to help run your metabolism and improve blood sugar and insulin functioning*	Follow the manufacturer's label instructions for dosage. Most good multivitamins and minerals require 2 to 4 capsules or tablets a day to obtain adequate doses.
Purified fish oil (EPA/DHA)	*Acts as an anti-inflammatory, insulin- and blood sugar–balancing, heart-disease-preventing, brain-boosting supplement*	2 to 4 grams a day
Vitamin D$_3$	*Helps insulin function*	2,000 to 4,000 units a day
L-carnitine	*Assists with fat burning for fuel*	300 to 400 milligrams twice a day
Coenzyme Q10 (antioxidant)	*Helps to optimize energy production and supports heart health*	30 milligrams twice a day
PGX fiber (superfiber)	*Slows blood sugar and insulin spikes and can also cut cravings and promote weight loss*	2.5 to 5 grams just before every meal with a large glass of filtered water. Can be taken as powder or softgels.
Magnesium glycinate (relaxation mineral)	*Helps to reduce anxiety, improve sleep, assist blood sugar control, cure muscle cramps, and help with constipation*	100 to 150 milligrams (2 to 3 capsules once or twice a day)

(continued)

Supplement	Benefits	Daily Dosage
Probiotics	*Helps normalize your gut flora*	10 to 20 billion CFU (colony-forming units)
MCT oil (superfat from coconut oil)	*Speeds up your metabolism, improves liver function, and fuels your brain*	1 to 2 tablespoons a day
Electrolytes (E-lyte) (combination of electrolytes and salt); optional	*Helps with proper tissue hydration and makes you feel amazing*	1 to 2 capfuls a day
Potato starch; optional (I recommend Bob's Red Mill Unmodified Potato Starch, available at most local health-food stores)	*A form of "resistant starch" that helps balance your blood sugar and feed the good gut bugs, both of which help with weight loss*	Build up to 1 to 2 tablespoons in 8 ounces of filtered water twice a day

A TYPICAL DAY ON *EAT FAT, GET THIN*

Now that you've stocked your kitchen with nutritious foods and the right tools and supplements, you're ready to start the twenty-one-day plan. The full plan can be found in my book *Eat Fat, Get Thin*, but here's a snapshot:

Morning

- Begin the day with 30 minutes of movement (walking or other exercise)
- Before breakfast, take 2.5 to 5 grams of the PGX fiber (1 to 2 packets or ½ to 1 scoop of the powder in 10 ounces of filtered water, or 3 to 6 capsules)
- Take your supplements with breakfast
- Take your MCT oil or add your MCT oil to your coffee or smoothie
- Make and eat your smoothie or breakfast
- Optional: Have a midmorning snack (you can find snack recipes beginning on page 88)

- Drink water (at least 8 glasses throughout the day); use at least 1 capful of E-lyte in 8 ounces of filtered water twice a day to help with proper hydration

Afternoon

- Before lunch, take 2.5 to 5 grams of the PGX fiber
- Eat lunch
- Optional: Have a midafternoon snack
- Drink water (at least 8 glasses throughout the day)

Evening

- Before dinner, take 2.5 to 5 grams of the PGX fiber
- Eat dinner
- Optional: Have 1 tablespoon of potato starch in water before bed
- Get 7 to 8 hours of quality sleep

It's as easy as that. But I promise, three simple weeks can drastically change your life.

3

Tips, Tips, and More Tips

I've put together a few tips that will enhance your three-week experience and beyond, on everything from grocery shopping to cooking with fats to preparing meals for the kids. I use these tricks to get the most out of my food and my time, and they have made me feel less stressed about putting healthy meals on the table every day.

TIP 1: HOW TO MAKE THE MOST OF YOUR FATS

I want to touch briefly on cooking with fats since they are the main focus of this plan. Fat is complicated. Unlike sugar, different fats interact with your body in different ways. For example, trans fats increase inflammation, while omega-3 fats reduce inflammation. Some fats destabilize when heated, so they become toxic to the body when cooked, while other fats remain stable at higher temperatures and can actually enhance the vitamin and mineral assimilation in different ingredients. Here are a few easy tips that will maximize the amount of nutrition you get out of your food.

Oils

Knowing which oils to use, and what to use them for, is the key to experiencing their benefits.

Coconut oil, sesame oil, avocado oil, and ghee are best for higher-heat cooking, as they have a higher smoke point and do not become toxic as quickly as other oils when exposed to heat. Olive oil is best for low-heat cooking or, used raw, for dressing salads. Macadamia oil and walnut oil also are wonderful raw and make great dressings.

With all oils, always choose organic, unrefined, cold-pressed, or expeller-pressed. Be sure to do your research, and don't be afraid to contact the company directly to ensure that the product is truly cold-pressed. Organic production prohibits GMOs and the use of hexanes for extraction in oils.

Store oils in dark, not clear, bottles and keep in a cool, dark place away from light and heat. Don't store oils on kitchen counters or next to the stove because they will oxidize or turn rancid. Always close the lid tightly, and immediately store oils after using them because oxygen contributes to rancidity. Oils go bad over a span of months depending on type. That's why it is so important to purchase only the amount you will use within two months. You can see a list of my favorite brands of oils at www .eatfatgetthin.com/resources.

Animal Fats

Grass-fed and pasture-raised animals live in cleaner, healthier, and more sustainable environments compared with animals raised on feedlots. That's why I always recommend buying grass-fed *and* grass-finished beef (meaning the animal has been raised on grass for its entire life) whenever possible.

The meat and dairy from feedlot-raised animals have less nutritional benefit for us and contain harmful additives and contaminants such as antibiotics, hormones, and pesticides. Animals in feedlots are fed diets of genetically modified (GMO) grains, corn, barley, and soybeans to speed up weight gain. Studies have linked the consumption of genetically modified food (including meat) to serious health risks in humans, such as infertility, immunity problems, faster aging, improper insulin function, and changes in vital organs, including the gastrointestinal system. Feedlot animals are often given antibiotics and growth hormones, and when we eat feedlot meat, we are also exposed to these.

When animals suffer, the whole planet suffers. It's an undisputed fact that healthy and happy animals make for healthy meat. I like to get my meats from local farms so I can talk to the farmers about the way the animals were raised and see their living conditions and food with my own eyes if possible. It is important to choose your meats wisely to receive their full nourishing benefits and take responsibility for the lives of the animals that provide the food we consume.

Fish and Seafood

Fish and seafood are the absolute best sources of complete omega-3 fatty acids, EPA and DHA, but toxic mercury levels make it vital to choose fish from the best possible source. I personally suffered from mercury toxicity as a result of growing up on tuna fish sandwiches, eating a ton of sushi, and having a mouth full of amalgam fillings. I felt tired and weak all the time. I suffered from depression, anxiety, digestive problems, and other debilitating symptoms. Mercury toxicity is one of the most prevalent ailments that I see in my practice. Avoiding fish high in this heavy metal is of the utmost importance.

According to the Environmental Working Group, the best sources of omega-3 fish that also contain the lowest levels of mercury are wild salmon, sardines, mussels, rainbow trout, herring, anchovies, and Atlantic mackerel. The fish we should avoid are king mackerel, lobster, marlin, tuna, halibut, Chilean sea bass, orange roughy, shark, swordfish, and tilefish. To avoid toxic exposure, we should choose wild and high-quality fish sources whenever possible.

Nuts and Seeds

Everyone who knows me knows that I am nuts for nuts and seeds! They make the perfect snack or topping for your salads, and they are filled with healthy fats and vitamins and minerals that can improve your hormones, your brain health, and your heart health. However, nuts and seeds also contain phytates, which bind to important minerals, such as iron, zinc, magnesium, and calcium, and limit absorption of these minerals from the digestive tract. These minerals play a critical role in preventing diabetes and obesity, and a deficiency in them is often seen with type 2 diabetes.

Soaking and rinsing raw nuts and seeds effectively reduces the phytates and enzyme inhibitors.

Soaking is a pretty simple process: Soak raw nuts or seeds in warm salt water (1 tablespoon of salt for 4 cups of nuts or seeds) overnight or for up to twenty-four hours. Make sure the nuts and seeds are fully submerged in the water. Once they are finished soaking, rinse them off thoroughly. It's important to let them dry fully so they don't mold. Lay them out in the sun or spread them on a pan and place in the oven on a warm setting, no more than 120°F. With a dehydrator, you can set the heat setting to no more than 108°F and still preserve most nutrients. Dehydrate or leave in oven for twelve to twenty-four hours.

TIP 2: HOW TO EAT WELL ON A BUDGET

When I was in residency, I had to support a wife and two kids on $27,000 a year. I have met with families all over the world with limited finances, and they were still able to eat well on a budget. It is absolutely possible with a little bit of planning, and you're still going to be able to enjoy delicious and flavorful meals, I promise. Here are my eating-for-less strategies:

1. Ditch the processed and packaged foods! Good news: You will already be doing this on the *Eat Fat, Get Thin* Plan. In terms of price per nutrient density, fruits and veggies are way less expensive than packaged foods. I also recommend avoiding "healthy" packaged foods. These are the boxes and bags that line the shelves at your health-food store. They are usually overpriced and often full of sugar, even if it is organic cane sugar. Plus, if you take a look at the ingredients, you'll find you can quite often just as easily make these foods at home. Kale chips require a few spices, some oil, and an oven. While you're at it, skip the coffee lines, too. Even buying just one coffee a day adds up fast, and combining all those convenience-food purchases, you might be shocked at how much you're spending and how easy it is to make healthier alternatives in your own

kitchen. Write down how much money you spend on little things every day, expenses you could avoid and would save you money for real food.

2. Hit the discount stores. Trader Joe's and Costco carry organic products, often for cheaper than at other grocery stores. Try Thrive Market, an online store carrying the same healthy home and food products found at Whole Foods but at 25 to 50 percent off the retail price. Receive a one-month free trial plus 15 percent off your first order if you sign up at this link: www.thrivemarket.com/efgt.

3. Learn to love and prepare at least five to ten basic recipes. Keep ingredients for these recipes around at all times so that you can quickly make them when you're in a bind or low on time. You can also save money by freezing meats and leftovers so they don't go bad.

4. Buy in bulk and stock up when you see a sale on your favorite storable foods. Don't forget, you can freeze a lot of foods or ingredients that you won't use right away. People who live in rural areas often find that a chest freezer is a wise investment if trips to the grocery store are infrequent.

5. Check out the guide from the Environmental Working Group called Good Food on a Tight Budget (www.ewg.org).

TIP 3: HOW TO GROCERY SHOP WITH EASE

Shopping for healthy and delicious foods can be done just about anywhere. You don't have to have access to farmers' markets, gourmet-food stores, or even health-food stores. You can go to your regular grocery store and usually find what you need, and it doesn't take very long either. Also, don't be afraid to ask your local grocery store to carry specific items for you. The more people ask, the more likely the store is to bring new items in, and even if you're the only person asking for it, you might be pleasantly surprised at how accommodating the store is. So if you don't see organic almond butter or organic produce, ask for it! In fact, Walmart is the biggest seller of organic produce in the country.

The first step is to make a shopping list. This obviously saves you from wandering the aisles aimlessly and subsequently purchasing junk food on impulse. The second step is to stick to the outside aisles, or, more specifically, the produce section, for your main ingredients, and remember, when selecting beef or meat, choose grass-fed, hormone-free, or organic, when possible. Next, load up on the following essentials, which will make cooking (and healthy choices) easier:

- Extra-virgin olive oil
- Extra-virgin coconut oil
- Other favorite oils, such as walnut, sesame, flax, and avocado
- Nuts, such as walnuts, almonds, pecans, and macadamia
- Seeds, such as hemp, chia, flax, pumpkin, and sesame
- Unsweetened nut milk
- Almond flour and coconut flour
- Canned full-fat coconut milk, unsweetened
- Kalamata olives
- Apple cider vinegar
- Balsamic vinegar
- Bone broth (homemade or low-sodium chicken or vegetable stock)
- Dijon mustard
- Sea salt
- Freshly ground black pepper
- Seasonings and spices, such as cayenne, cinnamon, chili powder, cumin, curry powder, garlic powder, oregano, onion powder, paprika, parsley, rosemary, sage, thyme, and turmeric
- Wheat-free tamari (low-sodium)

Most of these staples can be found at big discount stores, but some might not be available at your grocery store, or they may be unreasonably priced. That's when online shopping can be very useful. Thrive Market is my favorite online market to buy wholesome foods at wholesale prices. They carry every single staple that I've mentioned, plus plenty more. If online shopping feels easier to you, head over to www.thrivemarket.com /efgt for more information.

TIP 4: HOW TO SAVE TIME

When you're short on time, it is incredible how a little bit of strategic planning goes a very long way.

Frozen fruits and vegetables are key time-savers. I like to stock my freezer with frozen berries, vegetables, grass-fed beef, and wild salmon.

I also recommend buying prewashed and precut veggies (organic, of course) if you're short on time. This will help you cut down on time spent prepping in the kitchen. But by learning a few simple knife skills you can slice your own and save money. And it's more fun! Carefully chosen canned, jarred, and boxed foods are another great option. Watch for those tricky additives when you're buying them, but overall, things like nut butters, coconut milk, canned sardines, wild Alaskan salmon, artichokes, and roasted red peppers make great additions to salads. Any packaged foods should contain only a few ingredients, and ones that you recognize such as tomatoes, water, and salt.

Pick a day when you have some free time and do a little planning for your week. If you have any prep work that can be done in advance, this would be the time to do it. Put on your favorite music or podcast, and wash, cut, and store your vegetables, ideally in glass containers, or even freeze them. Make some batches of sauces or dips that will keep for a few days, and create a meal plan for the week. This helps with grocery shopping and with sticking to a budget. Also, try to make at least double the amount of any recipe that you know you'll want to have leftovers of or incorporate into another meal. For example, grass-fed burgers and hand-cut roasted sweet potato fries one night can easily become shepherd's pie the next night.

There are many days you may want to cook without a recipe. In fact, that is what I do over 90 percent of the time for simple, delicious, healthy food. Here are easy ways to cook your veggies and meats:

To Steam Veggies

Pour 1 cup of filtered water in the bottom of a saucepan and bring it to a boil over high heat. Place a steaming rack or basket over the boiling water. Chop your vegetables and place them in the steaming rack or basket, cover, and let them cook for 4 to 8 minutes, depending on the denseness of the vegetable.

To Blanch Veggies

Simply submerge your vegetables in boiling water and then turn down the heat while they soften.

To Sauté Veggies

Add 1 tablespoon of coconut oil, ghee, or expeller-pressed sesame oil to a sauté pan. After the oil is hot, add the vegetables, cooking them for 1 to 2 minutes. More dense and tough vegetables such as cauliflower will need a little longer.

To Grill Veggies

Heat a grill pan or an outdoor gas grill and brush with a small amount of olive oil. Place the vegetables on the grill and cook, turning once, until browned.

To Roast Veggies

Preheat the oven to 425°F. Toss the vegetables with olive oil, butter, or coconut oil, and season with sea salt and pepper. Arrange in a layer on a baking sheet and roast until crispy and tender. Times will vary depending on the vegetable.

To Sauté, Grill, or Roast Meats

Follow the same instructions for veggies, but always use a meat thermometer to assess internal temperature. Always insert in the thickest part of the meat for accuracy. The following guide provides temperatures at which different meats are considered done.

Steak: 130°F to 135°F for medium rare; 140°F to 145°F for medium
Fish: 145°F
Chicken: 160°F to 165°F
Ground beef: 165°F

TIP 5: HOW TO EAT OUTSIDE OF THE HOME

If you're invited to a party, have no fear; there are ways to enjoy yourself while staying on track. First things first, never skip meals. If you feel nervous about the food being served, eat before you arrive so you feel satiated and confident about staying away from junk foods. When people ask me why I am not indulging at a party, I tell them that I'm there for the people, not the food. No one argues with that, and no one can possibly feel insulted by it!

Once you arrive, find the vegetables and dips (as there is almost always at least one of these at every gathering), so if you want to munch on something, you have some pretty healthy options. Volunteering to bring something to every gathering you attend is a surefire way to guarantee there's food there you can eat. There are plenty of dips and sides in this book that everyone can enjoy (beginning on page 88). Try your best to avoid alcohol, as it's toxic and sugary and can lead you down a slippery slope of bad choices. Instead, bring or ask for sparkling water with lemon or lime. After your three-week program, you can enjoy your favorite drink from time to time.

Eating at a restaurant is a bit more manageable, as most restaurants are very accommodating to dietary needs. If possible, try to choose the restaurant yourself instead of leaving it up to someone else. That way you can control the types of foods you'll be enjoying. When I go to a restaurant with questionable entrées, I focus on the side dishes. There are often plenty of vegetable options, and there's nothing wrong with getting several sides as your entrée. You can always ask for a basic chicken or fish dish, or salad with a side of avocado, topped with olive oil and vinegar instead of sugary, creamy dressings. The most important piece of advice: Do the best you can and focus on the company you are with, not the food.

TIP 6: HOW TO EAT WITH KIDS

Studies show the family that eats together stays together. Given the opportunity, most kids love to play in the kitchen and are always open to trying new foods as a family. Picky eaters are definitely out there, but keep in mind that it sometimes takes kids a few times of trying something new before they decide whether or not they like it. Also keep in mind that making a big deal out of a picky eater's refusal of a particular food only makes it more likely to occur. No drama. Choose your battles and let kids develop their own palates without stress.

Make mealtime a pleasant, relaxed, joyful experience (good for digestion!) and involve your kids in the cooking process. When they are able to help create a meal, they are more likely to eat it. Food should not be used for punishment or reward. This creates a dangerous emotional relationship with food that can carry into adulthood.

Also, set realistic boundaries about food choices and mealtimes. If you want to raise a healthy eater, my recommendation is to not create separate meals for the kids and adults. Once children are old enough to chew solids, expose them to a variety of foods, including the foods that you eat every day. As long as the meal or food is not super spicy, kids should generally be eating all the healthy and varied foods their parents eat. America is the only country with kids' menus and foods. In Japan, kids eat raw fish, and in parts of Africa kids eat reptiles, not chicken nuggets or macaroni and cheese.

If your child has a sophisticated palate, he or she might enjoy all the meals in this book, but the following are sure to be winners with all kids:*

Breakfast

Walnut Pancakes with Blueberries (page 82)
Strawberry-Mint Chia Pudding (page 87)
Creamy Strawberry and Greens Smoothie (page 61)
Banana-Raspberry-Coconut Smoothie (page 65)

Snacks, Sides, Soups

Deviled Eggs (page 102)
Classic Guacamole (page 93)
Sweet Potato Soup with Coconut and Ginger (page 136)

---

* Be aware of allergens. Many of these recipes contain coconut, nuts, and nut milk.

Lunch or Dinner

Turkey Burgers with Peppers and Onions (page 220)
"Spaghetti" and Meatballs with Tomato Sauce (page 226)
Tempeh, Vegetable, and Kelp Noodle Stir-Fry (page 171)

Dessert

Raspberry-Coconut Ice Cream (page 262)
Spiced Sweet Potato Quick Bread (page 251)
No-Bake Walnut Brownies (page 259)

TIP 7: HOW TO SNACK

The number one thing that can derail your plans is getting caught in a food emergency. When your blood sugar drops, everything, even Twinkies, can start to look like a good option. Thinking that you can use willpower to maneuver your way out of these situations is not realistic. You need to be prepared for moments like this, especially when you're away from your healthy home base. Snacking is perfectly fine on this program, and even though you might not need snacks because increased fat cuts cravings, I still recommend keeping certain foods on hand in case of an emergency.

The key to smart snacking is to stick to protein, fats, or low-glycemic carbs. The reason this works is because sugary processed carbs are addictive, and we don't know when to stop eating them, but fats and proteins are satiating, and when you've had enough, your body tells you instantly. Do you ever find yourself overeating broccoli? I didn't think so. We've included plenty of snack recipes starting on page 88, but if you are looking for items to purchase and take on the go, these are my recommendations:

- Canned wild salmon or sardines
- Jerky (bison, grass-fed beef, salmon, or turkey)
- Nuts and seeds (almonds, walnuts, pecans, macadamia nuts, and pumpkin seeds)

- Nut butter, single-serving packets (almond, pecan, macadamia)
- Coconut butter (you can buy it in convenient single-serving packets)

For short trips and to take to the office or school:

- Hard-boiled omega-3 eggs
- Cut-up carrots, cucumbers, peppers, and celery in ziplock baggies (pair with guacamole)
- ½ cup mixed berries in a small bag
- Sometimes I love to cut open an avocado, sprinkle a little salt or wheat-free tamari or balsamic vinegar on top of it, and eat it with a spoon.

I've teamed up with Thrive Market to create an Emergency Fat Snack Pack that is filled with my favorite snacks, including canned wild salmon, grass-fed jerky, nuts and seeds, and almond butter squeeze packs. When you're traveling or running out of time, this snack pack will prevent you from running into a food emergency. Visit www.thrivemarket.com/efgt for more information.

TIP 8: HOW TO SWAP GOOD FOR BAD

Cravings for your old favorites may pop up from time to time, but there are always healthier alternatives. So try these instead of those.

Instead of	*Try*
Bread	Spiced Sweet Potato Quick Bread (page 251)
Chips	Nuts (almonds, cashews, macadamia nuts, etc.) Dehydrated or roasted veggies such as kale, carrots, zucchini
Soda	Sparkling water with a little bit of lemon or lime
Pasta	Kelp noodles, zucchini noodles, spaghetti squash

(continued)

Instead of	Try
Yogurt	Strawberry-Mint Chia Pudding (page 87), coconut yogurt
Candy	Mixed berries
Mashed potatoes	Butternut squash, sweet potato mash, cauliflower mash
Cheese	Nutritional yeast
Peanut butter	Almond butter, cashew butter, coconut butter

TIP 9: HOW TO DEAL WITH YOUR HEALING CRISIS

It is not uncommon for the body to have a strong reaction when you stop feeding it the processed foods and chemicals it is accustomed to. This is called a healing crisis or a detox crisis.

Food companies have chemically engineered their foods to be biologically addictive, and the result is that many people are hooked on processed junk food. Ridding your system of these toxic foods can cause some uncomfortable reactions, such as achy, flu-like feelings, irritability, nausea, headaches, sleep difficulties, and constipation. The good news is that these symptoms usually pass within forty-eight hours. So first and foremost, give your body time to adjust. If possible, start the twenty-one-day plan on a weekend or when you have some time off to lay a bit lower than usual for a day or two if you need to.

A strong negative reaction to a cleanse or detox is more common with calorie-restrictive programs such as juice cleanses, so that's why I always recommend food-based programs to avoid detoxing too quickly. Prep days or transition weeks are also helpful to get your body adjusted to the types of foods you'll be eating. If the *Eat Fat, Get Thin* Plan is drastically different from your normal diet, I recommend giving yourself a few days to experiment with the approved foods and get used to things slowly, before adding in supplements.

Another way to ease healing-crisis symptoms is to increase circulation and flush the toxins out of your body by going for a walk outside, taking a sauna, or getting a massage. It's very important to make sure your bowels are moving. If you're backed up, toxins will remain in the body and you'll feel pretty awful. To combat constipation, first and foremost, stay hydrated. Try sprinkling ground flaxseeds into your salads or smoothies. Magnesium citrate also helps with bowels, sleep, and stress. If none of those strategies work, you can take an herbal laxative such as cascara, senna, or rhubarb. De-stress however possible, because stress is incredibly constipating.

Other options to ease your detox include getting plenty of rest. Make your bedroom a tranquil haven and your bed a place for sleep or romance only. Try to avoid screen time and eating for at least one to two hours before bed.

Going low-carb very quickly can cause a drop in energy for some people. If you feel fatigued for more than a few days, contact one of our coaches at www.drhyman.com. Most of the time, adding salt or E-lyte electrolytes can help as you are getting off the carbs. When you drop your insulin level you will drop a lot of retained fluid and salt along with it, so adding more salt helps prevent you from feeling dizzy and weak.

If your detox symptoms persist for a longer period of time, it may mean that something deeper is going on, and in that case I recommend the help of a Functional Medicine practitioner, but one to three days of adjustment is common for most people.

4

Transitioning to the Pegan Diet

After twenty-one days, you have the option of staying on the *Eat Fat, Get Thin* Plan or transitioning to what I call the Pegan Diet. After years of experimenting with different diets (vegan, vegetarian, Paleo, low-fat, low-carb) and seeing thousands of patients, I've finally landed on this one. It has left me feeling better than ever and has transformed the lives of people all over the world.

What is Pegan? Well, a Pegan Diet combines the best of the Paleo and vegan diets, which have a lot more in common than you might think. A healthy vegan diet and a healthy Paleo diet place an emphasis on real, whole, fresh food that is sustainably raised and is rich in vitamins, minerals, and phytonutrients, while being low in sugar, refined carbs, and processed foods and ingredients. Essentially, the Pegan Diet is all about eating real food.

In order to determine whether or not you should transition, I recommend heading over to www.eatfatgetthin.com/resources and taking the recommended quizzes, tests, and measurements before and after the twenty-one days. There are two quizzes in particular (the Feel Like Crap Quiz and the Carbohydrate Intolerance Quiz) that will show you your toxicity levels before you start the program and after. I highly recommend taking these quizzes so that you can monitor your progress and decide whether or not to stay on the *Eat Fat, Get Thin* Plan or transition.

Here are the steps to transitioning to a Pegan Diet:

1. Add in beans and gluten-free grains such as black rice, quinoa, and buckwheat in moderation. See what works for your unique body.

For some, these foods might cause inflammation, a spike in insulin and blood sugar, and digestive issues. So it's best to test these foods out slowly to see how your body reacts to them. Do you feel good or do you feel bloated? Does your skin break out? How are your energy levels? Does any sort of negative reaction follow the consumption of these foods?

2. Continue to eat the right fats. Stay away from inflammatory (processed vegetable) fats and continue to focus on the good fats, such as nuts and seeds, wild fatty fish, avocados, and coconut oil.

3. Eat mostly plants—plenty of low-glycemic vegetables and fruits. These should make up 75 percent of your diet and your plate.

4. Power up with protein. Again, protein is essential for muscle synthesis and appetite control, and it speeds up your metabolism.

5. Stay away from dairy (except for grass-fed butter), because it's inflammatory and filled with hormones.

6. Stay away from gluten. If you are not gluten sensitive, then consider it an occasional treat. Try small amounts of non-gluten grains such as black rice, quinoa, and buckwheat.

7. Continue with the daily supplements and thirty minutes of movement (that you find enjoyable) each day.

8. I'll let you in on a little secret. I don't eat a perfect diet 100 percent of the time. When traveling or socializing, we're all occasionally tempted with "junk" foods. Think of sugar and flour as recreational drugs. Once you've achieved all of your health goals and weight-loss goals, you can indulge in these "recreational treats" occasionally without guilt. (Eating these foods and then punishing yourself with guilt is dangerous for your emotional and physical health, so make sure you skip the self-reproach.) I've included some of my favorite dessert recipes for just these occasions (page 250).

You'll see Pegan recipes throughout this book. Just look for "Pegan Diet" underneath the recipe title. If you're on the twenty-one-day *Eat Fat, Get Thin* Plan, skip these recipes for now.

The Pegan Diet Food Pyramid

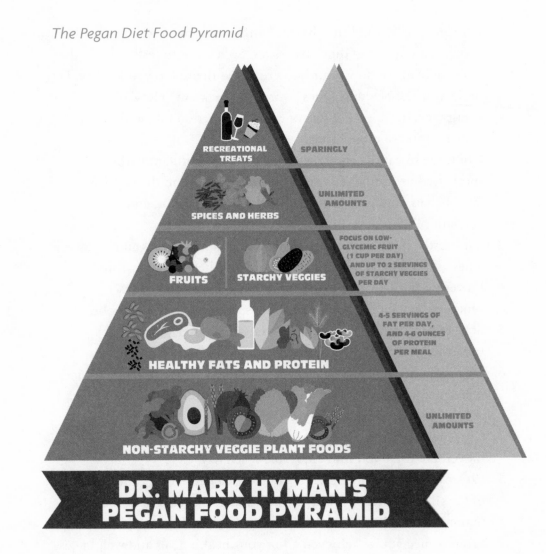

PART II

THE RECIPES

We have the power to transform our food industry and the health of the world. This transformation starts with you and what you put into your shopping carts, stock your home with, and serve on your kitchen table. It starts with what you eat every single day.

I believe we can vote with our dollars. Every time we purchase packaged, processed, GMO foods, we vote to keep ourselves sick and our planet sick. We also tell the corporations that's what we want. Every time we fill our kitchens with beautiful, real, whole, fresh foods and support our small local farms, we vote to keep ourselves and our planet healthy, and we send a loud and clear message to those same corporations.

Reconnecting with cooking and my kitchen has been one of the most transformative experiences of my life. Cooking has brought my family closer together. It has made me healthier, given me more energy and new goals, and created a new joy that I look forward to every mealtime. I believe that everyone is capable of achieving this joy by using food as medicine.

I am so thrilled to have teamed up with my friend Chef Frank Giglio to present these mouthwatering yet simple recipes that I hope will bring you as much pleasure as they bring me. Now you have all the tools you need. Let's get cooking!

Remember that all recipes that say "Pegan Diet" underneath the title are to be used after the twenty-one-day plan. All other recipes can be enjoyed at any time.

5

Smoothies and Beverages

BASIC NUT MILK

Makes: 4 cups
(strained)

Prep time:
2 minutes, plus
12 to 24 hours
for soaking

Store-bought nut milks often contain fillers and synthetic vitamins, so my rec-ommendation is to make your own. It's much easier than you might think. Just remember to soak the nuts overnight to soften them so that they blend more easily. Soaking also unlocks nutrients, making them easier to absorb and digest.

- 1 cup raw nuts (such as almonds, hazelnuts, walnuts, or Brazil nuts)
- 4 cups filtered water, plus water for soaking

Place the nuts in a glass container and add enough filtered water to cover the almonds by about 2 inches. Cover and refrigerate for at least 12 hours or for up to 24 hours.

Drain the nuts. Combine the nuts and the 4 cups filtered water in a blender. Begin blending on low speed, slowly increase the speed to high, and blend on high speed for 1 to 1½ minutes.

You can use the nut milk as is, or for a smoother consistency, strain the mixture through a nut-milk bag (available at most natural-food stores and online) into a large bowl; squeeze the bag to extract as much milk as possible from the pulp.

Transfer the nut milk to an airtight container and refrigerate for up to 3 days. Stir well or shake before using.

Nutritional analysis per serving (1 cup strained almond milk): *Calories: 128, Fat: 11.2 g, Saturated Fat: 0.8 g, Cholesterol: 0 mg, Fiber: 2.4 g, Protein: 4.8 g, Carbohydrates: 4.8 g, Sodium: 0 mg*

COCONUT MILK

Makes: 4 cups

Prep time:
5 minutes

Coconut milk is my favorite dairy-free alternative, especially for creating delicious smoothies and curries. It contains MCT oils, which can support heart health and help build muscle, and those are just a couple of its benefits. Full-fat coconut milk straight from the can is often too thick for smoothies, so if you're looking for a lighter flavor and consistency, try this recipe.

- 1 (13.5-ounce) can full-fat coconut milk
- 2¼ cups filtered water

Combine the coconut milk and filtered water in a glass container. Stir until well blended or cover with a tight-fitting lid and shake vigorously. Refrigerate, covered, for up to 5 days.

Nutritional analysis per serving (1 cup): *Calories: 202, Fat: 20 g, Saturated Fat: 19 g, Cholesterol: 0 mg, Fiber: 0 g, Protein: 0 g, Carbohydrates: 3 g, Sodium: 25 mg*

COCONUT-ACAI SMOOTHIE

Serves: 1

Prep time:
5 minutes

PEGAN DIET

Often considered a superfood, acai berries are known for their antioxidant benefits. Acai bowls—a puree of the berries topped with an assortment of fruits and nuts—have become popular breakfast meals. In this recipe, the frozen acai puree is blended with coconut to create a rich, flavorful, nutrient-dense smoothie.

- 1 (90-gram) pack frozen acai, cut into small chunks
- 2 tablespoons chopped raw shelled pistachios
- 1 date, pitted
- 2 teaspoons fresh lemon juice
- 1¼ cups Coconut Milk (page 55)
- ½ teaspoon vanilla powder

Combine all the ingredients in a blender and blend on high speed until smooth and creamy, about 45 seconds. Drink immediately.

Nutritional analysis per serving: Calories: 336, Fat: 17 g, Saturated Fat: 7 g, Cholesterol: 5 mg, Fiber: 6 g, Protein: 6 g, Carbohydrates: 44 g, Sodium: 15 mg

MANGO-COCONUT SMOOTHIE

PEGAN DIET

This tropical-flavored smoothie is one of my go-to blends, especially in the summer. It's enhanced with nutrient- and protein-rich hemp seeds and with creamy coconut butter, making it a satiating breakfast choice.

- 1 cup frozen mango chunks
- 1½ cups coconut water (or unsweetened nut milk or filtered water)
- 2 tablespoons hemp seeds
- 2 tablespoons coconut butter

Combine all the ingredients in a blender and blend on high speed until smooth and creamy, about 45 seconds. Drink immediately.

Nutritional analysis per serving: *Calories: 562, Fat: 30 g, Saturated Fat: 18 g, Cholesterol: 0 mg, Fiber: 12 g, Protein: 11 g, Carbohydrates: 76 g, Sodium: 111 mg*

Mixed Berry-Coconut Smoothie

Serves: 1

Prep time:
5 minutes

Coconut milk is a nutritious and creamy source of high-quality fat, making it the perfect choice for satiating smoothies like this one. This quick and easy smoothie made with frozen berries is an excellent choice for breakfast or a snack. For added richness, freeze coconut milk in an ice-cube tray and use the frozen cubes in place of regular ice cubes.

- 1½ cups frozen mixed berries
- 1 cup full-fat coconut milk, chilled
- 1 cup ice cubes
- 1 teaspoon ground cinnamon
- ½ teaspoon alcohol-free, gluten-free pure vanilla extract (or ¼ teaspoon unsweetened vanilla powder)
- grated zest of 1 lemon

Combine all the ingredients in a blender and blend on high speed until smooth and creamy, about 45 seconds. Drink immediately.

Nutritional analysis per serving: Calories: 327, Fat: 24 g, Saturated Fat: 22 g, Cholesterol: 0 mg, Fiber: 4 g, Protein: 1 g, Carbohydrates: 24 g, Sodium: 47 mg

CHERRY BOMB SMOOTHIE

PEGAN DIET

Serves: 1

Prep time: 5 minutes

Talk about an antioxidant powerhouse! This morning beverage includes a trifecta of healing spices: cinnamon, nutmeg, and ginger. Combined with fatty hazelnuts and antioxidants from cherries, this smoothie will jump-start your day in just the right way.

- 1½ cups unsweetened Hazelnut Milk (page 54)
- ¾ cup frozen pitted sweet cherries
- ½ teaspoon ground cinnamon
- ½ teaspoon freshly grated nutmeg
- ½ teaspoon ground ginger
- ½ teaspoon alcohol-free, gluten-free pure vanilla extract (or ¼ teaspoon unsweetened vanilla powder)
- 1 tablespoon coconut butter

Combine all the ingredients in a blender and blend on high speed until smooth and creamy, about 45 seconds. Drink immediately.

Nutritional analysis per serving: *Calories: 479, Fat: 21 g, Saturated Fat: 8 g, Cholesterol: 0 mg, Fiber: 5 g, Protein: 8 g, Carbohydrates: 68 g, Sodium: 6 mg*

Cherry-Hemp Smoothie

Serves: 1

Prep time:
5 minutes

PEGAN DIET

Hemp seeds are a great source of protein, magnesium, zinc, iron, and phosphorus. Needless to say, they are an excellent addition to your diet and are easy to incorporate into smoothies and salads. This five-ingredient smoothie is super easy to whip together first thing in the morning or after a workout.

- 1½ cups unsweetened almond milk
- ½ cup frozen pitted sweet cherries
- 2 tablespoons hemp seeds
- 1 tablespoon hemp oil
- ½ teaspoon ground ginger

Combine all the ingredients in a blender and blend on high speed until smooth and creamy, about 45 seconds. Drink immediately.

Nutritional analysis per serving: *Calories: 387, Fat: 25 g, Saturated Fat: 2 g, Cholesterol: 0 mg, Fiber: 5 g, Protein: 8 g, Carbohydrates: 29 g, Sodium: 2 mg*

CREAMY STRAWBERRY AND GREENS SMOOTHIE

Arugula is one of the best nutrient-dense types of leafy greens. It's a great source of phytochemicals and antioxidants that have been known to combat cancer. Throwing a handful of greens into your smoothie is an easy way to get more nutrients into your diet.

Serves: 1

Prep time: 5 minutes

- 1½ cups unsweetened Hazelnut or Almond Milk (page 54)
- ½ avocado, pitted and peeled
- 1 cup frozen strawberries
- 1 handful baby arugula (about 1 packed cup)
- 1 tablespoon coconut oil, melted

Combine all the ingredients in a blender and blend on high speed until smooth and creamy, about 45 seconds. Drink immediately.

Nutritional analysis per serving: *Calories: 544, Fat: 31 g, Saturated Fat: 15 g, Cholesterol: 0 mg, Fiber: 21 g, Protein: 9 g, Carbohydrates: 42 g, Sodium: 248 mg*

OMEGA-3 GREEN SMOOTHIE

Fats + protein + slow carbs is my go-to formula for creating fulfilling meals that keep me satisfied for hours. This smoothie has that combination, and every single ingredient contains powerful nutrition that will leave you feeling vibrant. I usually start my day with this blend or some variation of it.

- 1½ cups coconut water, chilled
- 1 tablespoon hemp oil
- 1 tablespoon chia seeds
- 1 cup frozen strawberries or raspberries
- ½ avocado, pitted and peeled
- 1 large handful baby spinach
- 1 tablespoon toasted shredded coconut, for garnish (optional)

Combine all the ingredients in a blender and blend on high speed until smooth and creamy, about 45 seconds. Top with the toasted coconut, if using, and drink immediately.

Nutritional analysis per serving: Calories: 530, Fat: 34 g, Saturated Fat: 6 g, Cholesterol: 0 mg, Fiber: 22 g, Protein: 7 g, Carbohydrates: 41 g, Sodium: 368 mg

Minted Green Smoothie with Raspberries

If you're looking to pack a lot of nutrition into a quick, portable meal, look no further than green smoothies. They're perfect for kids who don't like the taste of greens. Here, peppermint tea imparts a fresh, herbal note.

- 1 peppermint tea bag
- 1 cup frozen raspberries
- 2 handfuls baby spinach
- 4 ice cubes
- 2 tablespoons hemp seeds
- 1 tablespoon MCT oil

Place the tea bag in a ½-pint Mason jar or other heatproof glass container and pour in 1½ cups boiling water. Cover and let steep for 10 minutes, then remove and discard the tea bag. Refrigerate the tea until cold.

Combine the chilled tea, raspberries, spinach, ice, hemp seeds, and MCT oil in a blender and blend on high speed until smooth and creamy, about 45 seconds. Drink immediately.

Nutritional analysis per serving: *Calories: 395, Fat: 25 g, Saturated Fat: 15 g, Cholesterol: 0 mg, Fiber: 9 g, Protein: 8 g, Carbohydrates: 19 g, Sodium: 11 mg*

Peachy Green Smoothie

Serves: 1

Prep time:
5 minutes

PEGAN DIET

A complete protein, spirulina is high in chlorophyll, B vitamins, and an assortment of minerals. Don't let the blue-green color scare you off! This unique smoothie will surprise you with its delicious flavor.

- 2 cups unsweetened Almond Milk (page 54), chilled
- 1 cup frozen sliced peaches
- 2 tablespoons almond butter
- 1 tablespoon chia seeds
- 2 teaspoons spirulina

Combine all the ingredients in a blender and blend on high speed until smooth and creamy, about 45 seconds. Drink immediately.

Nutritional analysis per serving: *Calories: 441, Fat: 28 g, Saturated Fat: 2 g, Cholesterol: 0 mg, Fiber: 10 g, Protein: 12 g, Carbohydrates: 40 g, Sodium: 379 mg*

BANANA-RASPBERRY-COCONUT SMOOTHIE

Serves: 1

Prep time:
5 minutes

PEGAN DIET

I think of this smoothie as a drinkable treat. The frozen banana creates a creamy texture that kids will love. As a bonus, the drink is filled with delicious and nutritious high-quality fats.

- 1 cup coconut water (or filtered water), chilled
- 1 banana, peeled and frozen
- ¾ cup frozen raspberries
- 2 tablespoons coconut butter
- 1 tablespoon coconut oil
- 2 cups baby spinach

Combine all the ingredients in a blender and blend on high speed until smooth and creamy, about 45 seconds. Drink immediately.

Nutritional analysis per serving: Calories: 625, Fat: 36 g, Saturated Fat: 30 g, Cholesterol: 0 mg, Fiber: 26 g, Protein: 5 g, Carbohydrates: 48 g, Sodium: 248 mg

CHOCOLATE-RASPBERRY SMOOTHIE

Serves: 1

Prep time:
5 minutes

The classic combination of chocolate and raspberry makes for a double whammy of antioxidants! (Cacao contains large amounts of *both* antioxidants and magnesium.) A little touch of ghee boosts the fat content and enhances this delectable treat of a smoothie.

- 1½ cups unsweetened Nut Milk (page 54), chilled
- ¾ cup frozen raspberries
- 1 heaping tablespoon cacao powder
- 1 tablespoon Ghee (page 279)
- 2 dates, pitted (optional, use during Pegan Diet)
- 1 teaspoon unsweetened vanilla powder

Combine all the ingredients in a blender and blend on high speed until smooth and creamy, about 45 seconds. Drink immediately.

Nutritional analysis per serving: Calories: 379, Fat: 20 g, Saturated Fat: 9 g, Cholesterol: 0 mg, Fiber: 11 g, Protein: 7 g, Carbohydrates: 50 g, Sodium: 253 mg

PUMPKIN PIE BULLETPROOF COFFEE

It's Bulletproof Coffee with a seasonal twist. Spiked with the superfat MCT, this beverage will warm you up and keep you satisfied for hours.

- 1½ cups freshly brewed coffee, hot
- 1 tablespoon unsalted, grass-fed butter
- 2 teaspoons MCT oil
- 2 teaspoons pumpkin pie spice
- 1 teaspoon alcohol-free, gluten-free pure vanilla extract
- 1 tablespoon maple syrup (optional)

Combine all the ingredients, including maple syrup, if using, in a blender and blend on high speed until frothy, about 45 seconds. Drink immediately.

Nutritional analysis per serving: Calories: 349, Fat: 33 g, Saturated Fat: 24 g, Cholesterol: 61 mg, Fiber: 1 g, Protein: 0 g, Carbohydrates: 18 g, Sodium: 21 mg

Serves: 1

Prep time: 10 minutes (including coffee-brewing time)

REISHI MUSHROOM–COFFEE ELIXIR

Serves: 1

Prep time:
5 minutes

Reishi mushrooms have an array of health benefits, including immune-system support. If you haven't experimented with reishi mushrooms, I highly recommend trying this hot drink—it's a comforting and tasty introduction. Mushroom extracts and capsules are readily available through online merchants and at most health-food stores.

- 1½ cups freshly brewed coffee, hot
- 1 tablespoon Ghee (page 279) or coconut oil
- ½ teaspoon alcohol-free, gluten-free pure vanilla extract
- 6 (1,000-milligram) reishi mushroom capsules

Combine the coffee, ghee, and vanilla in a blender. Open each reishi capsule and empty the contents into the blender; discard the capsules. Blend on high speed until combined, about 30 seconds. Drink immediately.

Nutritional analysis per serving: Calories: 200, Fat: 11 g, Saturated Fat: 7 g, Cholesterol: 30 mg, Fiber: 0 g, Protein: 0 g, Carbohydrates: 0 g, Sodium: 107 mg

6

Eggs and Other Breakfast Dishes

Slow-Fried Eggs with Onion and Basil

Serves: 4

Prep time:
5 minutes

Cook time:
8 minutes

By frying eggs over gentle heat on a bed of onion slices, you can create soft, creamy eggs that taste almost as if they have been poached. Add some fragrant basil and you have an aromatic dish that will wake up the whole family.

- 3 tablespoons extra-virgin olive oil
- 2 teaspoons unsalted, grass-fed butter
- 1 small red onion, sliced into very thin rounds
- 4 large eggs
- 1 teaspoon sea salt
- ¼ teaspoon freshly ground black pepper
- ¼ cup fresh basil leaves, torn into small pieces

In an 8-inch skillet, warm 1 tablespoon of the olive oil and the butter over medium heat until shimmering. Fan out the onion slices in an even layer and cook without stirring until slightly softened, about 2 minutes. Using a metal spatula, flip the onion slices, then crack an egg into each quadrant of the pan, on top of the onion. Cook for 2 minutes, then drizzle the eggs with 1 tablespoon of the remaining olive oil and sprinkle with the salt and pepper. Partially cover the pan and cook until the egg whites are set but the yolks are still runny, 3 to 4 minutes.

Drizzle the eggs with the remaining 1 tablespoon olive oil. Transfer 1 egg with some of the onion slices to each of 4 plates, sprinkle with basil, and serve.

Nutritional analysis per serving: Calories: 200, Fat: 19 g, Saturated Fat: 5 g, Cholesterol: 190 mg, Fiber: 0 g, Protein: 6 g, Carbohydrates: 1 g, Sodium: 670 mg

BUTTERY BROCCOLI AND SPINACH WITH FRIED EGGS

Serves: 4

Prep time:
15 minutes

Cook time:
15 minutes

This dish is the perfect way to power up before a long day. It includes my favorite combination of greens, fat, and protein and makes for a comforting, hearty breakfast. I recommend cooking the eggs sunny-side up so that the yolks, when broken, act as a sauce for the vegetables.

- 8 ounces broccoli (1¼ cups), stems peeled and cut into ¼-inch-thick rounds, florets cut into bite-size pieces
- 1½ tablespoons Ghee (page 279)
- ½ yellow onion, sliced thin
- 2 garlic cloves, minced
- 4 cups baby spinach
- ½ teaspoon sea salt
- ¼ teaspoon freshly ground black pepper
- 1 tablespoon unsalted, grass-fed butter
- 4 large eggs
- 2 avocados, pitted, peeled, and cut into slices

In a medium saucepan, bring 4 cups of filtered water to a boil over high heat. Add the broccoli. Use a spatula to keep the broccoli submerged in the water and cook until tender, 2 to 3 minutes. Using a slotted spoon, transfer the broccoli to a plate.

In a large sauté pan, warm the ghee over medium–high heat until melted. Add the onion and cook, stirring occasionally, until softened, 3 to 4 minutes. Stir in the garlic and cook until fragrant, about 30 seconds. Add the spinach and the cooked broccoli and stir to incorporate. Sprinkle the salt and the pepper on top and stir to combine. Remove from the heat and cover to keep warm.

In an 8-inch skillet, warm the butter over medium heat until foaming. Carefully crack an egg into each quadrant of the pan and cook until the egg whites are fully set but the yolks are still runny, 3 to 4 minutes. (For over-easy eggs, use a metal spatula to gently flip each egg and cook for 1 minute.)

Divide the vegetable mixture among 4 plates, and top each portion with an egg. Garnish with the avocado slices, dividing them evenly, and serve.

Nutritional analysis per serving: Calories: 290, Fat: 23 g, Saturated Fat: 7 g, Cholesterol: 187 mg, Fiber: 11 g, Protein: 12 g, Carbohydrates: 15 g, Sodium: 721 mg

POACHED EGGS WITH HOLLANDAISE

Serves: 4

Prep time: 10 minutes

Cook time: 30 minutes

Hollandaise, one of the five mother sauces in classic French cuisine, is simply an emulsion of egg yolks and melted butter. Here, hollandaise gets an upgrade, with ghee replacing the butter. Serve blanched asparagus or sautéed spinach alongside for a perfect brunch.

- 8 large eggs, plus 3 yolks
- ¾ cup Ghee (page 279), melted and kept warm
- ½ teaspoon sea salt
- 2 teaspoons fresh lemon juice
- ⅛ teaspoon cayenne pepper
- 2 tablespoons apple cider vinegar

Fill a large saucepan with 1 inch of water, bring to a simmer over medium heat, then reduce the heat to low.

In a medium heatproof bowl, combine the egg yolks and 1 teaspoon water and whisk until the yolks lighten in color, 1 to 2 minutes. Set the bowl over the simmering water in the saucepan (make sure the bottom of the bowl doesn't touch the water) and whisk constantly until the mixture is thick enough to coat the back of a spoon, 3 to 5 minutes.

Remove the bowl from the pan and gradually whisk in the warm ghee, drop by drop to start, then increased to a slow but steady stream. Add the salt, lemon juice, and cayenne and whisk to combine. Place the bowl back over the simmering water occasionally so the hollandaise stays warm until you are ready to serve, but be careful not to let it overheat or the sauce will break.

Fill a 2-quart pot with 2 inches of filtered water and bring to a simmer over medium heat. Stir in the vinegar. Crack each egg into a ramekin or teacup, then, one at a time, carefully slide the eggs into the water. Let the eggs cook undisturbed until the whites are just set but the yolks are still runny, 3 to 4 minutes.

Using a slotted spoon, place two poached eggs on each of 4 plates. Drizzle warm hollandaise over the top and serve.

Nutritional analysis per serving: *Calories: 588, Fat: 58 g, Saturated Fat: 31 g, Cholesterol: 508 mg, Fiber: 0 g, Protein: 14 g, Carbohydrates: 1 g, Sodium: 426 mg*

EGGS BAKED ON PORTOBELLO MUSHROOMS

Serves: 4

Prep time:
20 minutes

Cook time:
15 minutes

This is a fun recipe to make for breakfast or brunch guests. As they bake, the meaty mushroom caps soften and absorb the herbaceous pesto, so they're flavored throughout. Make sure not to overcook the eggs, as the runny yolks act as a sauce for the mushrooms.

- 4 large portobello mushrooms
- 2 tablespoons extra-virgin olive oil
- ½ cup Arugula Pesto (page 269)
- 4 large eggs
- 12 cherry tomatoes, cut in half

Preheat the oven to 350°F.

Remove and discard the stems from the mushrooms. Using a spoon, gently scrape away the gills from the underside of the mushroom caps. If the caps don't sit stably with the stemmed sides facing up, trim the rounded sides so that they do.

Place the caps stemmed side up in a 9- by 13-inch baking dish and drizzle them with the olive oil. Spread 2 tablespoons of the pesto on each cap, carefully crack an egg on top, and place 6 cherry tomato halves around each egg. Bake until the egg whites have set but the yolks are still a bit runny, 6 to 8 minutes.

Carefully transfer each egg-topped mushroom to a plate and serve.

Nutritional analysis per serving: Calories: 209, Fat: 16 g, Saturated Fat: 3 g, Cholesterol: 187 mg, Fiber: 3 g, Protein: 9 g, Carbohydrates: 6 g, Sodium: 158 mg

ITALIAN BREAKFAST SCRAMBLE

Serves: 4

Prep time:
15 minutes

Cook time:
10 minutes

Here's a delicious breakfast to enjoy in the summer, when tomatoes and zucchini are at the height of their season. Basil is rich in potassium and a good source of iron and vitamins A, C, and K. The addition of this powerful, aromatic herb will make you feel as though you're vacationing in Italy.

- 4 large eggs
- 1 teaspoon sea salt
- ¼ teaspoon freshly ground black pepper
- 2 tablespoons extra-virgin olive oil
- 1 zucchini, finely diced
- 1 small red onion, finely diced
- 2 garlic cloves, thinly sliced
- 8 cherry tomatoes, cut in half
- ¼ cup julienned fresh basil
- 1 tablespoon unsalted, grass-fed butter, at room temperature

In a bowl, whisk together the eggs, salt, and pepper.

In a large nonstick skillet, warm the olive oil over medium heat until shimmering. Add the zucchini and onion and cook, stirring occasionally, until softened, 2 to 3 minutes. Stir in the garlic and cook until fragrant, about 1 minute. Add the tomatoes and cook just until heated through, 3 to 4 minutes. Pour in the eggs and, using a wooden spoon, stir until the eggs form soft curds, about 3 minutes. Remove from the heat, fold in the basil and butter, and serve.

Nutritional analysis per serving: *Calories: 392, Fat: 15 g, Saturated Fat: 4 g, Cholesterol: 193 mg, Fiber: 4 g, Protein: 16 g, Carbohydrates: 53 g, Sodium: 533 mg*

Spicy Egg Scramble with Tomato and Avocado

Serves: 4

Prep time:
10 minutes

Cook time:
10 minutes

Switch up your egg breakfast with this spicy twist on basic scrambled eggs. Jalapeños contain capsaicin, an anti-inflammatory substance that has been shown to promote healthy weight loss. Feel free to turn up the heat or turn it down by using more or less jalapeño.

- 8 large eggs
- ¼ teaspoon sea salt
- ½ teaspoon freshly ground black pepper
- 2 tablespoons coconut oil
- 1 large red onion, thinly sliced
- 1 jalapeño, sliced into thin rounds
- 1 large tomato, roughly chopped
- 1 avocado, pitted, peeled, and sliced
- ¼ cup fresh cilantro leaves, roughly chopped

In a bowl, whisk together the eggs, salt, and pepper.

In a large nonstick skillet, warm the coconut oil over medium heat until shimmering. Add the onion and jalapeño and cook, stirring occasionally, until softened, 4 to 5 minutes. Pour in the eggs and, using a wooden spoon, stir until the eggs form soft curds, about 3 minutes.

Divide the eggs among 4 plates. Top with the tomato, avocado slices, and cilantro and serve.

Nutritional analysis per serving: Calories: 247, Fat: 21 g, Saturated Fat: 8 g, Cholesterol: 370 mg, Fiber: 4 g, Protein: 14 g, Carbohydrates: 11 g, Sodium: 293 mg

MUSHROOM AND EGG SCRAMBLE

Serves: 4

Prep time:
10 minutes

Cook time:
10 minutes

Mushrooms bring a meaty, earthy quality to any dish. In this recipe, I opt for cremini mushrooms, or baby portobellos as they are sometimes called. If you're a fan of fungi, try experimenting with other varieties such as oyster and shiitake, or even with more unusual mushrooms such as black trumpet or lion's mane.

- 8 large eggs
- 3 scallions, thinly sliced
- 1 teaspoon sea salt
- 2 tablespoons coconut oil
- 4 cups cremini mushrooms, thinly sliced
- 2 avocados, pitted, peeled, and diced

In a bowl, whisk together the eggs, scallions, and salt.

In a large skillet, warm the coconut oil over medium-high heat until melted. Add the mushrooms and cook, stirring frequently, until softened and lightly browned, about 3 minutes. Pour in the eggs and, using a wooden spoon, stir until the eggs form soft curds, 2 to 3 minutes.

Divide the scramble among 4 plates. Top with the diced avocados and serve.

Nutritional analysis per serving: Calories: 296, Fat: 25 g, Saturated Fat: 10 g, Cholesterol: 185 mg, Fiber: 9 g, Protein: 9 g, Carbohydrates: 13 g, Sodium: 508 mg

Smoked Salmon and Asparagus Frittata

Serves: 4

Prep time:
15 minutes

Cook time:
35 minutes,
plus cooling
time

A frittata is one of my go-to dishes when I want a nutritious, satisfying meal without a lot of time-consuming or labor-intensive cooking. You can play around with the ingredients, changing the vegetables and seasonings to suit your taste. This combination is my favorite because it features two of the best sources of high-quality fat: coconut and salmon.

- 8 large eggs
- ½ cup full-fat coconut milk
- 2 tablespoons thinly sliced chives
- ½ teaspoon freshly ground black pepper
- 2 tablespoons coconut oil
- 1 yellow onion, chopped
- 2 garlic cloves, minced
- 1 bunch asparagus, trimmed and cut into 1-inch pieces
- 4 ounces smoked salmon, cut into ¼-inch pieces

Preheat the oven to 350°F.

In a bowl, whisk together the eggs, coconut milk, chives, and pepper.

In an 8-inch nonstick oven-safe skillet, warm the coconut oil over medium-high heat until shimmering. Add the onion and cook, stirring occasionally, until softened, 2 to 3 minutes. Stir in the garlic and cook until fragrant, about 1 minute. Add the asparagus and cook, stirring occasionally, until slightly softened, 2 to 3 minutes. Stir in the salmon, then pour in the egg mixture. Transfer the pan to the oven and cook until the center of the frittata is firm to the touch and the eggs are fully set (a toothpick inserted into the center should come out clean), about 20 minutes.

Allow the frittata to cool for 5 minutes, then carefully run a spatula around the edges and underneath it to loosen it from the pan. Slide the frittata onto a plate, cut into four wedges, and serve.

Nutritional analysis per serving: *Calories: 347, Fat: 26 g, Saturated Fat: 15 g, Cholesterol: 370 mg, Fiber: 3 g, Protein: 22 g, Carbohydrates: 6 g, Sodium: 514 mg*

KIMCHI AND SPINACH FRITTATA

Serves: 4

Prep time:
5 minutes

Cook time:
25 minutes

This simple frittata features two very important ingredients: spinach and kimchi. Spinach is a vitamin- and mineral-dense supergreen, and kimchi (Korean fermented vegetables) is a probiotic-rich food that can improve gut function.

- 6 large eggs
- ½ cup full-fat coconut milk
- ½ teaspoon sea salt
- ¼ teaspoon freshly ground black pepper
- 1 tablespoon unsalted, grass-fed butter
- 6 cups baby spinach
- ½ cup drained kimchi, roughly chopped

Preheat the oven to 350°F.

In a bowl, whisk together the eggs, coconut milk, salt, and pepper.

In an 8-inch oven-safe skillet, warm the butter over medium heat until foaming. Add the spinach and stir until wilted. Pour in the egg mixture, add the kimchi, and stir to evenly distribute. Transfer the pan to the oven and cook until the center of the frittata is firm to the touch and the eggs are fully set (a toothpick inserted into the center should come out clean), about 20 minutes.

Allow the frittata to cool for 5 minutes, then carefully run a spatula around the edges and underneath it to loosen it from the pan. Slide the frittata onto a plate, cut into four wedges, and serve hot, warm, or at room temperature.

Nutritional analysis per serving: *Calories: 249, Fat: 16 g, Saturated Fat: 9 g, Cholesterol: 285 mg, Fiber: 7 g, Protein: 22 g, Carbohydrates: 14 g, Sodium: 726 mg*

GARLICKY BEEF AND SPINACH FRITTATA

Serves: 4

Prep time:
10 minutes

Cook time:
25 minutes,
plus cooling
time

This hearty breakfast is rich in healthy fats from the beef, eggs, and ghee. Garlic, known for its anti-inflammatory and medicinal properties, adds a delectable flavor and aroma to the frittata.

- 8 large eggs
- 2 teaspoons sea salt
- 2 tablespoons Ghee (page 279)
- 1 large yellow onion, finely diced
- 3 garlic cloves, minced
- 8 ounces beef flank steak, cut across the grain into thin strips
- ½ cup baby spinach

Preheat the oven to 350°F.

In a bowl, whisk together the eggs and salt.

In an 8-inch nonstick oven-safe skillet, warm the ghee over medium heat until melted. Add the onion and cook, stirring occasionally, until softened, 2 to 3 minutes. Stir in the garlic and cook until fragrant, about 1 minute. Stir in the beef and cook until the slices are medium-rare, about 2 minutes. Add the spinach and stir constantly until the spinach is wilted. Pour in the eggs and stir to evenly distribute. Transfer the pan to the oven and cook until the center of the frittata is firm to the touch and the eggs are fully set (a toothpick inserted into the center should come out clean), about 20 minutes.

Allow the frittata to cool for 5 minutes, then carefully run a spatula around the edges and underneath it to loosen it from the pan. Slide the frittata onto a plate, cut into four wedges, and serve.

Nutritional analysis per serving: Calories: 667, Fat: 24 g, Saturated Fat: 10 g, Cholesterol: 408 mg, Fiber: 6 g, Protein: 40 g, Carbohydrates: 80 g, Sodium: 1096 mg

SOUTHWESTERN TOFU SCRAMBLE

Serves: 4

Prep time:
20 minutes

Cook time:
15 minutes

Tofu lovers, this one's for you! I encourage my community to choose only GMO-free soy products and avoid all genetically modified soy foods because of the health risks they pose. This hearty, flavorful scramble can be enjoyed by vegans, vegetarians, and omnivores alike.

- 1 pound non-GMO firm tofu
- 2 tablespoons extra-virgin olive oil
- 1 small yellow onion, finely diced
- 1 red bell pepper, seeded and finely diced
- 1 green bell pepper, seeded and finely diced
- 1 summer squash, finely diced
- 2 garlic cloves, minced
- 2 teaspoons chili powder
- 1 teaspoon ground cumin
- 1 teaspoon sea salt
- 1 large tomato, roughly chopped
- ½ cup fresh cilantro leaves, roughly chopped
- ¼ cup toasted pumpkin seeds

Use a clean towel to squeeze excess water out of the tofu, and then use a fork or knife to crumble the tofu into bite-size pieces.

In a large skillet, warm the olive oil over medium-high heat until shimmering. Add the onion, bell peppers, summer squash, and garlic and cook, stirring occasionally, until the vegetables are slightly softened, about 3 minutes. Stir in the tofu and cook until warmed through, about 3 minutes. Sprinkle in the chili powder, cumin, and salt and stir to combine. Add the tomato and cook, stirring occasionally, until the tomato has broken down and any moisture has evaporated, 4 to 5 minutes.

Divide the scramble among 4 plates. Top with the cilantro and pumpkin seeds and serve.

Nutritional analysis per serving: *Calories: 468, Fat: 16 g, Saturated Fat: 2 g, Cholesterol: 0 mg, Fiber: 9 g, Protein: 24 g, Carbohydrates: 64 g, Sodium: 763 mg*

Walnut Pancakes with Blueberries

Serves: 4

Prep time:
5 minutes

Cook time:
15 minutes

Who said that being healthy means giving up pancakes? These delicious breakfast treats are grain-free, sugar-free, and dairy-free, so they're completely guilt-free, too! The whole family will love them.

- 6 large eggs
- 1½ cups unsweetened almond milk
- 1 tablespoon fresh lemon juice
- 2 teaspoons alcohol-free, gluten-free pure vanilla extract
- 1 cup coconut flour
- 1 cup arrowroot
- 2 teaspoons ground cinnamon
- 1 teaspoon baking powder
- 1 teaspoon baking soda
- ½ teaspoon sea salt
- ½ cup toasted walnuts, roughly chopped
- coconut oil, for cooking the pancakes
- 1 cup blueberries

In a large bowl, whisk the eggs. Add the almond milk, lemon juice, and vanilla, and whisk until well blended.

In a separate bowl, mix together the coconut flour, arrowroot, cinnamon, baking powder, baking soda, and salt. While whisking continuously, add the flour mixture ¼ cup at a time to the egg mixture. Gently fold in the walnuts.

In a large skillet, warm 1 tablespoon coconut oil over medium heat. When the skillet is hot, ladle batter into 3-inch rounds (about ¼ cup each) into the skillet; form as many pancakes as will comfortably fit. Cook the pancakes until bubbles appear on the surface, 2 to 3 minutes. Use a metal spatula to flip each pancake and cook for 2 to 3 more minutes. Transfer the pancakes to a wire rack. Add more coconut oil to the skillet and repeat to cook the remaining batter.

Divide the pancakes among 4 plates. Top with the blueberries and serve.

Nutritional analysis per serving: Calories: 315, Fat: 15 g, Saturated Fat: 11 g, Cholesterol: 139 mg, Fiber: 11.5 g, Protein: 9 g, Carbohydrates: 35.5 g, Sodium: 293 mg

Buckwheat Porridge

PEGAN DIET

Most people think buckwheat is a grain, but it is actually a seed. I like to use buckwheat not only because it is rich in fiber, but also because it contains protein, can improve digestion, and is a good source of powerful antioxidants. This hearty, nutty-tasting porridge is a great gluten-free alternative to oatmeal.

- 1 cup buckwheat groats
- 3 cups unsweetened almond milk
- 1 cinnamon stick
- 1 teaspoon alcohol-free, gluten-free pure vanilla extract
- ⅛ teaspoon sea salt
- ¼ cup maple syrup
- 1 cup mixed berries
- 2 tablespoons unsweetened shredded coconut, toasted

In a saucepan, combine the buckwheat groats, almond milk, cinnamon, vanilla, and salt. Cover and cook over medium heat, stirring occasionally, until the buckwheat is tender and has absorbed the almond milk, about 20 minutes. Remove and discard the cinnamon stick.

Divide the porridge among 4 bowls. Drizzle each portion with 1 tablespoon of the maple syrup, top with ¼ cup of the berries, and sprinkle with 1½ teaspoons of the toasted coconut. Serve.

Nutritional analysis per serving: Calories: 186, Fat: 5 g, Saturated Fat: 2 g, Cholesterol: 0 mg, Fiber: 4 g, Protein: 3 g, Carbohydrates: 33 g, Sodium: 426 mg

SPROUTED BUCKWHEAT MUESLI

PEGAN DIET

Makes: 6 cups

Prep time:
10 minutes
(plus overnight)

For those mornings when you're looking for a hearty, egg-free meal, look no further than this muesli. The buckwheat, nuts, and seeds in this recipe are soaked for easier digestion. You can tailor the muesli to suit your taste—switch it up by using different nuts and seeds and even different fruits. Feel free to experiment.

- 2 cups buckwheat groats
- 1 cup raw pecans
- ½ cup raw walnuts
- ½ cup raw pumpkin seeds
- ½ cup shelled raw sunflower seeds
- 1 cup unsweetened shredded coconut
- 2 crisp, tart apples, grated down to the cores
- 2 teaspoons ground cinnamon
- 4 cups unsweetened Nut Milk (page 54)
- ¼ cup maple syrup (optional)

Put the buckwheat groats in a bowl and cover with 4 cups filtered water. Let soak for 2 hours at room temperature.

Drain the buckwheat in a colander and rinse well. Transfer to a shallow container, cover with a clean kitchen towel, and let sit at room temperature until the groats begin to sprout, at least 8 hours or up to overnight. Rinse and drain well.

While the buckwheat soaks, in a bowl, combine the pecans, walnuts, pumpkin seeds, and sunflower seeds. Cover with about 2 inches of filtered water and let soak at room temperature for 2 to 4 hours. Drain and rinse.

In a large bowl, combine the sprouted buckwheat, the soaked nuts and seeds, the coconut, the grated apples, and the cinnamon and stir to combine.

Divide the muesli among 4 serving bowls and pour 1 cup of the nut milk into each bowl. Drizzle 1 tablespoon maple syrup, if using, over each portion and serve.

Nutritional analysis per serving (1 cup): Calories: 578, Fat: 43 g, Saturated Fat: 13 g, Cholesterol: 0 mg, Fiber: 10 g, Protein: 13 g, Carbohydrates: 43 g, Sodium: 159 mg

STRAWBERRY-MINT CHIA PUDDING

Chia seed pudding is all the rage these days. It's not hard to see why. Chia is a great source of protein, fiber, and fats, and the neutral-tasting seeds absorb water easily and become gelatinous quickly. This is a pudding that's great for breakfast and for taking on the road for a midday snack.

Serves: 1

Prep time: 5 minutes, plus 30 minutes to 12 hours chilling time

- 1 cup unsweetened almond milk
- ½ cup frozen strawberries
- ¼ cup chia seeds
- ½ teaspoon alcohol-free, gluten-free pure vanilla extract
- 2 drops peppermint essential oil
- ½ cup fresh strawberries, hulled and sliced
- 1 tablespoon unsweetened coconut flakes

Combine the almond milk and strawberries in a blender and blend on high speed until smooth, about 30 seconds.

Place the chia seeds in a small mixing bowl, then stir in the strawberry–almond milk mixture, vanilla, and peppermint oil. Cover and refrigerate for at least 30 minutes or for up to 12 hours.

Top with the sliced fresh strawberries and coconut and serve.

Nutritional analysis per serving: *Calories: 517, Fat: 30 g, Saturated Fat: 17 g, Cholesterol: 0 mg, Fiber: 21 g, Protein: 9 g, Carbohydrates: 42 g, Sodium: 248 mg*

7

Appetizers and Snacks

Coconut-Curry Cashews

Makes: 2 cups

Cook time:
35 minutes

Here, the spiciness of curry powder is offset by the natural sweetness of raisins. Cashews are one of my favorite nuts and a good source of copper, phosphorous, magnesium, manganese, and zinc, making this simple snack a nutritious way to nosh.

- ½ cup raisins
- 2 cups raw cashews
- 2 tablespoons unsweetened shredded coconut
- 1 tablespoon curry powder
- 1 teaspoon sea salt

Put the raisins in a small bowl and cover with ¾ cup boiling filtered water. Let soak for 30 minutes.

Preheat the oven to 275°F. Line a baking sheet with parchment paper.

Transfer the raisins and their soaking water to a blender and blend on high speed for about 45 seconds. The puree should have the consistency of a loose paste; if it's watery, pour it into a fine-mesh sieve set over a bowl and let the excess moisture drain off.

In a bowl, combine the raisin puree, cashews, coconut, curry powder, and salt and mix until well combined. Spread the mixture on the prepared baking sheet and bake, stirring every 10 to 15 minutes, until the cashews are golden brown, 25 to 30 minutes.

Allow the cashews to cool completely and serve right away or store in an airtight container at room temperature for up to 1 month.

Nutritional analysis per serving (½ cup): *Calories: 250, Fat: 13 g, Saturated Fat: 7 g, Cholesterol: 0 mg, Fiber: 2 g, Protein: 4 g, Carbohydrates: 34 g, Sodium: 448 mg*

HERB-ROASTED ALMONDS

Makes: 4 cups

Prep time:
10 minutes

Cook time:
40 minutes

Nutritious snacks like this one are essential for staying on course with healthful eating while traveling, when at work, or simply when out and about. Almonds are a great source of healthy fats that help keep you feeling full. They also contain powerful prebiotics, especially in the skins, that are food for the friendly bacteria in the gut.

- 1 pound raw almonds
- 2 tablespoons extra-virgin olive oil
- 1 tablespoon sea salt
- 1 (4-inch) sprig rosemary, leaves only, finely chopped
- 2 large sprigs thyme, leaves only, finely chopped
- 1 teaspoon onion powder
- ½ teaspoon garlic powder
- ½ teaspoon ground fennel seed
- ½ teaspoon freshly ground black pepper

Preheat the oven to 275°F. Line a baking sheet with parchment paper.

In a large bowl, combine all the ingredients and mix well. Spread the almonds in an even layer on the prepared baking sheet and bake, stirring every 15 minutes, until golden brown, 30 to 40 minutes.

Allow the almonds to cool completely and serve right away or store in an airtight container at room temperature for up to 1 month.

Nutritional analysis per serving (2 tablespoons): *Calories: 178, Fat: 16 g, Saturated Fat: 1 g, Cholesterol: 0 mg, Fiber: 3 g, Protein: 6 g, Carbohydrates: 6 g, Sodium: 420 mg*

AVOCADO HALVES WITH SPICY HEMP SALT

Serves: 4

Prep time:
5 minutes

In this simple recipe, already-delicious avocados get a flavor upgrade with seasoned salt. I like to make a big batch of this seasoning and store it in an airtight container. It's great for sprinkling on salads and can be used in place of regular salt in just about any recipe.

- 2 tablespoons hemp seeds
- 1 tablespoon nutritional yeast
- 1 teaspoon sea salt
- ½ teaspoon garlic powder
- ¼ teaspoon cayenne pepper
- 4 avocados, halved and pitted

In a small bowl, stir together the hemp seeds, nutritional yeast, salt, garlic powder, and cayenne.

Sprinkle the hemp salt evenly over the avocado halves. Serve with spoons for scooping the avocado flesh from the skin.

Nutritional analysis per serving: *Calories: 302, Fat: 26 g, Saturated Fat: 4 g, Cholesterol: 0 mg, Fiber: 12 g, Protein: 7 g, Carbohydrates: 19 g, Sodium: 574 mg*

Avocado and Vegetable Salsa

Makes: 4 cups

Prep time:
10 minutes

Most dips and salsas that you find at the grocery store are filled with preservatives, so I vote for homemade instead. This way, you're able to monitor what you're putting into your body. Here's a rich, delicious salsa that's also very versatile—serve it with crudités or flax crackers as a snack or appetizer, or offer it as an accompaniment to fish and other proteins.

- 3 avocados, pitted, peeled, and cut into ½-inch chunks
- 6 cherry tomatoes, cut in half
- 1 red bell pepper, seeded and finely diced
- 1 celery rib, finely diced
- 2 scallions, thinly sliced
- ¼ cup fresh parsley leaves, roughly chopped
- 2 tablespoons hemp seeds
- 2 tablespoons fresh lemon juice
- 3 tablespoons extra-virgin olive oil
- 1 teaspoon sea salt
- ¼ teaspoon freshly ground black pepper

In a large bowl, toss together all the ingredients until well mixed. Serve right away or cover and refrigerate for up to 2 hours.

Nutritional analysis per serving (1 cup): *Calories: 377, Fat: 35 g, Saturated Fat: 5 g, Cholesterol: 0 mg, Fiber: 11 g, Protein: 9 g, Carbohydrates: 16 g, Sodium: 456 mg*

CLASSIC GUACAMOLE

Makes: 2 cups

Prep time:
10 minutes

Everyone should have a good recipe for guacamole in their repertoire. There are no surprises here — this is the classic, crowd-pleasing dip.

- 2 large avocados, halved and pitted
- 1 small yellow onion, minced
- 1 jalapeño, seeded and minced
- ¼ cup packed fresh cilantro leaves, roughly chopped
- 1 teaspoon sea salt
- juice of 1 lime, plus more if needed
- 1 large tomato, coarsely chopped

Using a paring knife, make crosshatch cuts in the flesh of each avocado half, cutting to but not through the skin. Use a spoon to scoop the flesh from the skins and place it in a medium bowl. With a fork, roughly mash the avocado. Stir in the onion, jalapeño, cilantro, salt, and lime juice, then fold in the tomato. Transfer the guacamole to a bowl and serve right away, or squeeze additional lime juice on top to prevent oxidation, cover, and refrigerate for up to 4 hours.

Store any leftover guacamole in an airtight container in the refrigerator for up to two days. Add a little more lime juice and the pit from the avocado to prevent oxidation.

Nutritional analysis per serving (½ cup): *Calories: 202, Fat: 21 g, Saturated Fat: 3 g, Cholesterol: 110 mg, Fiber: 8 g, Protein: 3 g, Carbohydrates: 16 g, Sodium: 900 mg*

Almond Hummus

Makes: 3 cups

Prep time:
15 minutes, plus
soaking time

Here's a chickpea-free twist on hummus, made with raw almonds that have been soaked to render them more digestible. Use it as a dip, spread, or side dish, or in any way you'd use traditional hummus.

- 2 cups raw almonds
- ⅓ cup sesame seeds
- ½ cup fresh parsley leaves
- 2 teaspoons ground cumin
- 2 garlic cloves
- juice of 2 lemons
- 1 tablespoon sea salt
- ¼ cup extra-virgin olive oil

Put the almonds in a bowl and cover with 4 cups filtered water. Let soak for 8 hours or for up to 12 hours at room temperature.

Drain the almonds and rinse well.

Combine the almonds, sesame seeds, parsley, cumin, garlic, lemon juice, and salt in a food processor and pulse until roughly ground, 5 or 6 pulses. Scrape down the sides of the bowl. With the machine running, add the olive oil and ¼ cup filtered water in a steady stream and process until the mixture is creamy, about 1 minute.

Transfer the hummus to a bowl and serve right away or refrigerate in an airtight container for up to 4 days. Serve with endive, cucumbers, or other cut veggies.

Nutritional analysis per serving (¾ cup): *Calories: 338, Fat: 23 g, Saturated Fat: 2 g, Cholesterol: 0 mg, Fiber: 5 g, Protein: 11 g, Carbohydrates: 26 g, Sodium: 684 mg*

ROMESCO HUMMUS

Makes: about
3 cups

Prep time:
10 minutes

PEGAN DIET

Chickpeas, the main ingredient in hummus, are fibrous, nutritional beans. Beans can cause blood sugar to spike, so I don't recommend this dip during the *Eat Fat, Get Thin* twenty-one-day plan, but if you find that beans agree with you, you'll love this hummus with a flavorful twist.

- 2 (15-ounce) cans chickpeas, rinsed and drained
- 2 tablespoons fresh lemon juice
- ½ cup Pecan Romesco (page 270)
- ½ cup extra-virgin olive oil
- 2 teaspoons sea salt
- ¼ teaspoon freshly ground black pepper

In a food processor, pulse the chickpeas until coarsely but uniformly ground, 5 or 6 pulses. Scrape down the sides of the bowl, add the lemon juice and Romesco, and process until combined, about 30 seconds. With the machine running, add the olive oil in a slow, steady stream. Scrape down the bowl, add the salt and pepper, and process until well combined, about 1 minute.

Transfer to a bowl and serve right away or refrigerate in an airtight container for up to 4 days.

Nutritional analysis per serving (¾ cup): *Calories: 259, Fat: 21 g, Saturated Fat: 2 g, Cholesterol: 0 mg, Fiber: 6 g, Protein: 6 g, Carbohydrates: 19 g, Sodium: 916 mg*

ARTICHOKE DIP WITH CRUDITÉS

Makes: 4 cups

Prep time:
15 minutes

Artichoke dip is a family favorite that I make whenever we have guests over. Artichokes are underutilized but impressively nutritious veggies, and if you purchase them in cans (fresh artichokes require a lot of time-consuming prep, and canned are just as good for you), you'll find that they'll become regular items on your grocery list. In this dip, I use my favorite cheese replacement, nutritional yeast, instead of inflammatory cheese.

- 1 (15-ounce) can artichoke hearts, rinsed, drained, and roughly chopped
- 2 cups Homemade Mayonnaise (page 265)
- ½ cup packed fresh parsley leaves, roughly chopped
- 1 large sprig thyme, leaves only, finely chopped
- 2 tablespoons fresh lemon juice
- 2 tablespoons nutritional yeast
- 1 teaspoon sea salt
- 3 celery ribs, cut into 2-inch pieces
- 1 large carrot, scrubbed and cut into large matchsticks
- 1 small daikon radish, peeled and cut into ¼-inch rounds

In a large bowl, stir together the artichokes, mayonnaise, parsley, thyme, lemon juice, nutritional yeast, and salt. Transfer the dip to a bowl and serve with the celery and carrot sticks and the daikon rounds.

Store leftovers in an airtight container for up to four days.

Nutritional analysis per serving (½ cup): *Calories: 123, Fat: 0 g, Saturated Fat: 0 g, Cholesterol: 0 mg, Fiber: 3 g, Protein: 2 g, Carbohydrates: 6 g, Sodium: 440 mg*

"Cheesy" Sunflower Seed Dip

Makes: about 2 cups

Prep time: 5 minutes

In this recipe, vitamin E–rich sunflower seed butter is transformed into a dip that's perfect for cucumbers, bell peppers, and any other vegetables in your fridge. To change up the flavor, try adding a few tablespoons of fresh chopped herbs such as parsley, dill, and cilantro.

- 1 cup sunflower seed butter
- ¼ cup extra-virgin olive oil
- ¼ cup apple cider vinegar
- 2 tablespoons wheat-free tamari
- 3 tablespoons nutritional yeast
- 2 garlic cloves

Combine all the ingredients in a high-speed blender and add 2 tablespoons filtered water. Blend on high speed until smooth and creamy, about 1 minute. Transfer the dip to a bowl and serve right away or refrigerate in an airtight container for up to 4 days.

Nutritional analysis per serving (½ cup): *Calories: 272, Fat: 24 g, Saturated Fat: 2 g, Cholesterol: 0 mg, Fiber: 2 g, Protein: 7 g, Carbohydrates: 9 g, Sodium: 190 mg*

Creamy Horseradish Dip

Makes: about
1 cup

Prep time:
5 minutes

This simple dip works great with vegetable crudités or as a sauce for grilled steaks or rich, oily fish such as salmon and trout.

- 1 cup Homemade Mayonnaise (page 265)
- 2 tablespoons drained prepared horseradish
- 1 tablespoon apple cider vinegar
- sea salt

In a small bowl, stir together the mayonnaise, horseradish, and vinegar. Season to taste with salt. Serve right away or refrigerate in an airtight container for up to 1 week.

Nutritional analysis per serving (¼ cup): Calories: 99, Fat: 11 g, Saturated Fat: 1.75 g, Cholesterol: 5.5 mg, Fiber: 0 g, Protein: 0 g, Carbohydrates: 0.25 g, Sodium: 100 mg

TAHINI SPREAD WITH GARLIC-SHALLOT OIL AND PARSLEY

Tahini, a paste made from sesame seeds, is a staple in my pantry. I like to use it as a base for dressings and sauces. Here, I use it in a spread that's perfect with crudités and flax crackers.

- ½ cup extra-virgin olive oil
- 1 large shallot, sliced into thin rounds
- 3 garlic cloves, crushed
- 2 large sprigs thyme, leaves only, finely chopped
- 1½ cups tahini
- ½ cup parsley leaves, roughly chopped
- 2 tablespoons apple cider vinegar
- 2 teaspoons sea salt

Makes: about 2 cups

Prep time: 15 minutes

Cook time: 5 minutes

In a medium skillet over low heat, warm the olive oil, shallot, and garlic until the oil is infused with flavor, 5 to 6 minutes. Remove from the heat, stir in the thyme, and allow to cool completely.

In a medium bowl, stir together the tahini, parsley, vinegar, salt, and oil mixture. Serve right away or refrigerate in an airtight container for up to 1 week.

Nutritional analysis per serving (½ cup): *Calories: 262, Fat: 25 g, Saturated Fat: 3 g, Cholesterol: 0 mg, Fiber: 3 g, Protein: 5 g, Carbohydrates: 7 g, Sodium: 410 mg*

ROASTED PARSNIP AND ALMOND SPREAD WITH SUN-DRIED TOMATOES

Makes: 4 cups

Prep time:
10 minutes

Cook time:
30 minutes

Parsnips are an earthy, naturally sweet, and fiber-rich root vegetable that's particularly delicious when roasted. Serve this creamy spread as a snack or appetizer with roasted or raw vegetables or as an accompaniment to roasted or grilled meats.

- 1 pound parsnips, peeled and trimmed
- 1 cup unsalted roasted almonds
- 2 garlic cloves
- 6 olive oil–packed sun-dried tomatoes
- grated zest of 1 lemon
- 1 teaspoon dried thyme
- 1 teaspoon dried oregano
- 2 teaspoons sea salt
- ¼ teaspoon freshly ground black pepper

Preheat the oven to 325°F.

Place the parsnips in a 9- by 13-inch baking dish and pour in 1 cup filtered water. Cover the pan with aluminum foil and bake until the parsnips are tender, 25 to 30 minutes. Remove from the oven, transfer the parsnips to a cutting board, and allow to cool completely. Cut each parsnip into 4 to 6 pieces.

In a food processor, process the almonds and garlic until well ground, about 45 seconds. Scrape down the sides of the bowl and add the parsnips, sun-dried tomatoes, lemon zest, thyme, oregano, salt, and pepper. Process until the mixture is well pureed, about 1 minute.

Transfer the spread to a bowl and serve right away or refrigerate in an airtight container for up to 4 days.

Nutritional analysis per serving (1 cup): Calories: 330, Fat: 20 g, Saturated Fat: 2 g, Cholesterol: 0 mg, Fiber: 11 g, Protein: 10 g, Carbohydrates: 33 g, Sodium: 901 mg

WALNUT AND CARAMELIZED ONION PÂTÉ

Studies show that consuming healthy amounts of good fats, such as those in walnuts, improves brain function and mood and helps promote an overall sense of well-being. Here's a recipe that features walnuts for rich, savory flavor. Enjoy this delicious spread with roasted veggies or on flax crackers.

Makes: 3 cups

Prep time:
15 minutes

Cook time:
15 minutes

- 2 cups raw walnuts
- 1½ tablespoons Ghee (page 279)
- 1 large yellow onion, thinly sliced
- 3 garlic cloves
- 4 sprigs thyme, leaves only, finely chopped
- 2 teaspoons sea salt
- ¼ teaspoon freshly ground black pepper
- 1 tablespoon apple cider vinegar
- 3 tablespoons extra-virgin olive oil

Preheat the oven to 350°F.

Spread the walnuts on a baking sheet and toast, stirring occasionally, until golden brown, 8 to 10 minutes. Allow to cool to room temperature.

Meanwhile, in a medium skillet, warm the ghee over medium-high heat until melted. Add the onion and cook, stirring occasionally, until softened and golden brown, 10 to 12 minutes. Transfer to a plate and allow to cool to room temperature.

In a food processor, combine the toasted walnuts, garlic, thyme, salt, and pepper and pulse until the walnuts are roughly chopped, 6 to 7 pulses. Add the caramelized onion and vinegar and process until smooth, about 45 seconds. With the machine running, add the olive oil in a slow, steady stream and process until fully incorporated.

Transfer the pâté to a 1-quart glass jar. Serve right away or cover and refrigerate for up to 5 days.

Nutritional analysis per serving (¾ cup): *Calories: 535, Fat: 54 g, Saturated Fat: 8 g, Cholesterol: 13 mg, Fiber: 5 g, Protein: 10 g, Carbohydrates: 12 g, Sodium: 887 mg*

DEVILED EGGS

Makes: 24

Prep time:
15 minutes

Cook time:
15 minutes

After years of being vilified, eggs are now recognized as a great source of high-quality fat and protein. If you're looking for an easy-to-prepare, crowd-pleasing appetizer, look no further.

- 12 large eggs
- ½ cup loosely packed parsley leaves
- ¼ cup Homemade Mayonnaise (page 265)
- 1 tablespoon apple cider vinegar
- 2 teaspoons Dijon mustard
- 1½ teaspoons sea salt
- 1 teaspoon garlic powder
- ¼ teaspoon chipotle powder

Place the eggs in a large saucepan and cover with filtered water by about 1 inch. Bring to a boil over high heat and cook for 1 minute. Immediately remove the pan from the heat, cover, and let stand for 5 minutes. Meanwhile, fill a large bowl with ice water.

Pour off the water in the pan, then carefully transfer the eggs to the ice water. Let stand until completely cooled, then remove the eggs and wipe them dry.

Carefully crack and peel the eggs, then cut each egg in half lengthwise. Pop the yolks out into a food processor and set the whites in a single layer in a baking dish or on a serving platter. Add the parsley to the food processor and pulse until combined, about 3 pulses. Add the mayonnaise, vinegar, mustard, salt, garlic powder, and chipotle powder and process until thoroughly mixed, about 30 seconds.

Using a spoon or a pastry bag, fill the egg whites with the yolk mixture, dividing it evenly. Serve right away or refrigerate in an airtight container for up to 3 days.

Nutritional analysis per serving (4 halves): *Calories: 221, Fat: 15 g, Saturated Fat: 3 g, Cholesterol: 353 mg, Fiber: 1 g, Protein: 13 g, Carbohydrates: 4 g, Sodium: 320 mg*

DIY Nori Bites

Serves: 4

Prep time:
10 minutes,
plus soaking
time

Nori is a seaweed that we normally associate with sushi, but here it's a holder for a mix of nutritious fillings. This is a fun buffet-style snack that's also a great appetizer for a casual get-together.

- 2 cups pumpkin seeds
- 2 garlic cloves
- 2 celery ribs, cut into 1-inch pieces
- ¼ cup drained kimchi or sauerkraut
- ¼ cup extra-virgin olive oil
- ½ teaspoon sea salt
- ¼ cup fresh lemon juice
- 8 nori sheets, cut into quarters
- 2 cups sprouts (such as sunflower, buckwheat, or radish)
- 2 avocados, pitted, peeled, and sliced ¼ inch thick
- hot sauce, for serving (optional)

Put the pumpkin seeds in a bowl and cover with 4 cups filtered water. Let soak for 2 to 3 hours at room temperature. Drain and rinse well.

In a food processor, pulse the soaked pumpkin seeds, garlic, celery, and kimchi until combined, then process until crumbly, about 45 seconds. Scrape down the bowl, add the olive oil, salt, and lemon juice, and process until combined. With the machine running, slowly add up to ½ cup filtered water in a steady stream until the mixture is spreadable, with the consistency of thick nut butter. Transfer to a bowl.

To serve, set out the pumpkin seed mixture and the nori, sprouts, avocado, and hot sauce, if using. Have guests make their own nori bites: spread pumpkin seed mixture on a piece of nori, top with sprouts and avocado, and sprinkle on hot sauce, if desired.

Nutritional analysis per serving (8 pieces): *Calories: 593, Fat: 49 g, Saturated Fat: 4 g, Cholesterol: 0 mg, Fiber: 30 g, Protein: 20 g, Carbohydrates: 22.6 g, Sodium: 340 mg*

CRISPY TEMPEH TRIANGLES

Serves: 4

Prep time:
5 minutes

Cook time:
10 minutes

Tempeh is a fermented soybean product rich in protein, so it's a great alternative to meat. Fermentation makes the soy easier to digest and also increases its nutrition. These triangles are a yummy snack to pack in a lunch to take to work or school.

- 1 (8-ounce) block organic, GMO-free tempeh
- ¼ cup coconut oil
- 1 teaspoon sea salt

Cut the tempeh in half horizontally, then cut each half on the diagonal into quarters. You will have a total of 8 triangles.

In a large skillet, warm the coconut oil over medium-high heat until shimmering. Add the tempeh triangles in a single layer, sprinkle with ½ teaspoon of salt, and cook until browned and crisp, 3 to 4 minutes. Carefully flip each triangle, sprinkle with the remaining salt, and cook until the second sides are browned and crisp, about 2 minutes.

Transfer the tempeh to a paper towel–lined plate. Let cool for a minute or two, then serve.

Nutritional analysis per serving: Calories: 227, Fat: 20 g, Saturated Fat: 13 g, Cholesterol: 0 mg, Fiber: 0 g, Protein: 11 g, Carbohydrates: 5 g, Sodium: 565 mg

CHOPPED SARDINES ON CUCUMBER SLICES

Ounce for ounce, sardines are one of the best sources of the omega–3 fatty acids EPA and DHA, both of which have been shown to lower triglycerides and total cholesterol levels. This simple, flavorful snack offers great nourishment whenever you need a little energy boost. Be sure to look for sardines packed in olive oil.

Serves: 4

Prep time:
5 minutes

- 1 small cucumber, sliced into ¼-inch rounds
- 1 (4.37-ounce) can sardines packed in olive oil
- juice of ½ lemon, seeded
- 1 tablespoon fresh dill, roughly chopped
- 1 small shallot, minced
- ¼ teaspoon cayenne pepper

Arrange the cucumber slices on a plate.

Pour 2 tablespoons of the oil from the sardines into a small bowl. Roughly chop the sardines, then add them to the bowl with the oil. Squeeze in the juice from the lemon half and add the dill, shallot, and cayenne. Stir until combined.

Spoon the sardine mixture onto the cucumber slices, dividing it evenly, and serve.

Nutritional analysis per serving: *Calories: 58, Fat: 3 g, Saturated Fat: 1 g, Cholesterol: 17 mg, Fiber: 4 g, Protein: 4 g, Carbohydrates: 9 g, Sodium: 45 mg*

Roasted Bone Marrow

Serves: 4

Prep time:
2 minutes

Cook time:
15 minutes

Delicious, deeply nourishing bone marrow is a great source of omega-3 fatty acids, vitamins, and minerals. Roasted marrow can be spread on gluten-free crackers, stirred into soups, or folded into scrambled eggs. Or you can enjoy the rich, buttery texture and flavor on its own, with just a spoon.

- 2 pounds beef marrowbones

Preheat the oven to 450°F.

Place the marrowbones in a roasting pan. Roast until the bones are golden brown and the marrow is soft, about 15 minutes.

Scoop the marrow out of the bones and serve.

Nutritional analysis per serving (half of a bone): *Calories: 299, Fat: 20 g, Saturated Fat: 9 g, Cholesterol: 0 mg, Fiber: 0 g, Protein: 25 g, Carbohydrates: 2 g, Sodium: 315 mg*

8

Salads

Farmers' Market Salad with Miso Dressing

Serves: 4

Prep time: 20 minutes

There's nothing I love more than a salad made with ingredients fresh from the local farmers' market. Fruits and vegetables grown locally and harvested at the height of their season are loaded with phytochemicals, and they taste better, too! The flavorful miso dressing works well on almost any type of veggies, so feel free to use it on whatever looks great at your farmers' market.

- ½ cup extra-virgin olive oil
- 2 tablespoons soy-free miso
- 2 tablespoons red wine vinegar
- 2 tablespoons fresh lemon juice
- 1 large zucchini, trimmed
- 1 large yellow summer squash, trimmed
- 8 cups mixed greens
- 1 large cucumber, sliced into thin rounds
- 4 radishes, very thinly sliced
- 12 cherry tomatoes, cut in half
- 1 avocado, pitted, peeled, and cut into chunks
- ¼ cup toasted shelled sunflower seeds

To make the dressing, in a bowl, whisk together the olive oil, miso, vinegar, and lemon juice. Set aside.

Using a spiral vegetable slicer (aka spiralizer) fitted with the shredder blade, cut the zucchini and summer squash into spaghetti-size spirals. Use kitchen shears to cut the spirals into shorter lengths.

Divide the greens among 4 serving bowls. Top the greens with the zucchini and summer squash spirals and the cucumber, radishes, tomatoes, and avocado chunks, evenly dividing the ingredients.

Whisk the dressing to recombine, then drizzle it over the salads. Sprinkle each salad with 1 tablespoon of the sunflower seeds and serve.

Nutritional analysis per serving: *Calories: 442, Fat: 35 g, Saturated Fat: 5 g, Cholesterol: 0 mg, Fiber: 7 g, Protein: 6 g, Carbohydrates: 20 g, Sodium: 381 mg*

Arugula, Cucumber, and Avocado Salad with Raspberry-Coriander Vinaigrette

Serves: 4

Prep time: 20 minutes

This salad is simple, light, and refreshing, and it's perfect at the height of summer, when raspberries are in season. At other times of the year, the vinaigrette can be made with frozen raspberries that have been thawed. The salad will still be beautiful *and* delicious!

- 8 cups baby arugula
- 1 large cucumber, peeled and sliced into thin rounds
- 2 avocados, pitted, peeled, and cut into small chunks
- 1 cup raspberries
- ½ cup extra-virgin olive oil
- ¼ cup apple cider vinegar
- 1 teaspoon ground coriander
- 1 teaspoon sea salt
- ¼ teaspoon freshly ground black pepper
- 2 sprigs mint, leaves only, thinly sliced

Spread out the arugula on a large platter, and top with the cucumber slices and avocado chunks.

Combine the raspberries, olive oil, vinegar, coriander, salt, and pepper in a blender and blend on high speed until smooth, about 30 seconds. Pour the vinaigrette into a fine-mesh sieve set over a bowl and use a rubber spatula to push the puree through; discard the seeds in the sieve.

Drizzle the vinaigrette over the salad, sprinkle with the mint, and serve.

Nutritional analysis per serving: *Calories: 410, Fat: 38 g, Saturated Fat: 5 g, Cholesterol: 0 mg, Fiber: 8 g, Protein: 3 g, Carbohydrates: 18 g, Sodium: 665 mg*

Escarole and Grapefruit Salad with Sherry Vinaigrette

Serves: 4

Prep time: 15 minutes, plus time to tenderize

PEGAN DIET

Escarole is a hardy leafy green with a slightly bitter flavor. Bitterness is slowly being bred out of our vegetables, as many people don't find it to be a desirable trait, but bitter foods naturally detoxify the liver and stimulate the production of enzymes that help wake up the digestive system. Bitter notes also help balance out sweet, sour, and salty flavors.

- 2 grapefruits
- ¼ cup extra-virgin olive oil
- 2 tablespoons sherry vinegar
- 1 tablespoon Dijon mustard
- 1 small shallot, minced
- ½ teaspoon sea salt
- 1 large head escarole, core removed, leaves sliced very thin (8 cups)
- ½ cup toasted walnuts, coarsely chopped

Cut off the top and bottom of a grapefruit. Stand the grapefruit on a cut side and, using a sharp knife, cut away the rind and white pith in strips from top to bottom, following the contour of the fruit. Slide the knife blade along each side of the membrane dividing the sections of flesh to separate the sections into individual pieces. Repeat with the remaining grapefruit.

In a small bowl, whisk together the olive oil, vinegar, mustard, shallot, and salt.

Place the escarole in a large bowl, drizzle in the dressing, and use tongs to gently toss until the greens are evenly coated. Allow the greens to sit for 10 minutes to tenderize. Divide the escarole among 4 plates, sprinkle with the walnuts, and top with the grapefruit segments. Serve.

Nutritional analysis per serving: *Calories: 300, Fat: 24 g, Saturated Fat: 7 g, Cholesterol: 0 mg, Fiber: 4 g, Protein: 5 g, Carbohydrates: 22 g, Sodium: 330 mg*

SHAVED ASPARAGUS AND RADICCHIO SALAD

Serves: 4

Prep time: 20 minutes

Most people are familiar with roasted or steamed asparagus, but this springtime vegetable can also be enjoyed raw. The trick is to shave the stalks into thin, noodle-like slices so that they're tender and pleasing to eat. A sharp Y-shaped vegetable peeler is the best tool for the job.

- 1 bunch thick-stalk asparagus, trimmed
- 1 head radicchio, cored and thinly sliced
- ¼ cup pine nuts, toasted
- 3 tablespoons extra-virgin olive oil
- 2 tablespoons fresh lemon juice
- ½ teaspoon sea salt
- ¼ teaspoon freshly ground black pepper

Working one at a time, lay the asparagus spears on a cutting board and use a Y-shaped vegetable peeler to shave the asparagus from top to bottom, creating long, thin slices.

Place the shaved asparagus in a large bowl and add the radicchio, pine nuts, olive oil, lemon juice, salt, and pepper and gently toss to combine.

Divide the salad among 4 plates and serve.

Nutritional analysis per serving: *Calories: 177, Fat: 16 g, Saturated Fat: 2 g, Cholesterol: 0 mg, Fiber: 3 g, Protein: 5 g, Carbohydrates: 7 g, Sodium: 282 mg*

Super Green Salad

Serves: 4

Prep time: 20 minutes

Massaging olive oil and salt into kale gently wilts the leaves so that they taste lightly cooked. When you don't feel like doing much cooking on a hot summer day, this is a perfect, ultrahealthy, super-quick dish to prepare.

- 2 bunches curly kale, stemmed and torn into small pieces
- 3 tablespoons extra-virgin olive oil
- 1 teaspoon sea salt
- 1 orange (any kind, optional for Pegan Diet)
- 2 cups shredded red cabbage
- 8 ounces broccoli (1¼ cups), stems removed, florets cut into bite-size pieces
- 2 avocados, pitted, peeled, and cut into large chunks
- 3 tablespoons spirulina
- 2 tablespoons hemp seeds
- 2 tablespoons fresh lemon juice
- 1 teaspoon dried thyme
- 1 teaspoon dried oregano

In a large bowl, toss the kale with the olive oil and salt. Use your hands to gently massage the leaves, helping them to soften and wilt. Let stand for 5 minutes.

Meanwhile, cut off the top and bottom of the orange, if using. Stand the orange on a cut side and, using a sharp knife, cut away the rind and white pith in strips from top to bottom, following the contour of the fruit. Slide the knife blade along each side of the membrane dividing the sections of flesh to separate the sections into individual pieces.

Add the orange sections, cabbage, broccoli, avocado chunks, spirulina, hemp seeds, lemon juice, thyme, and oregano to the kale. Toss to combine and serve.

Nutritional analysis per serving: *Calories: 540, Fat: 37 g, Saturated Fat: 5 g, Cholesterol: 0 mg, Fiber: 25 g, Protein: 17 g, Carbohydrates: 44 g, Sodium: 728 mg*

HEARTY SPINACH SALAD

Serves: 4

Prep time:
10 minutes

Cook time:
15 minutes

As autumn approaches and the days grow colder, this salad becomes one of my favorites because it's so comforting and satisfying. It's also filled with some of my favorite sources of healthy fats, namely, olives, olive oil, eggs, and avocado. If you want to boost the protein content, add slices of grilled chicken, steak, or tofu.

- 4 large eggs
- 12 green beans, trimmed
- 1 tablespoon extra-virgin olive oil
- 1 cup baby spinach
- 1 avocado, pitted, peeled, and cut into chunks
- 1 small red onion, thinly sliced
- 1 cup pitted Kalamata olives
- about ½ cup Rosemary Vinaigrette (page 273)

Place the eggs in a saucepan and cover with filtered water by about 1 inch. Bring to a boil over high heat and cook for 1 minute. Immediately remove the pan from the heat, cover, and let stand for 5 minutes. Meanwhile, fill a large bowl with ice water.

Pour off the water in the pan, then carefully transfer the eggs to the ice water. Let stand until completely cooled, then remove the eggs and wipe them dry (keep the ice bath for the green beans). Crack and peel the eggs, then cut them in half lengthwise. Set the eggs aside.

In a saucepan, bring 4 cups filtered water to a simmer over medium-high heat. Add the green beans and cook until the beans are tender-crisp, about 3 minutes. Drain immediately and transfer the beans to the ice water to stop the cooking. Once the beans are chilled, drain again and transfer to a small bowl. Drizzle with the olive oil and toss to combine.

Divide the spinach among 4 plates and place 2 egg halves on each portion. Top with the green beans, avocado chunks, onion slices, and olives, evenly dividing each ingredient. Drizzle each salad with a couple of tablespoons of vinaigrette and serve.

Nutritional analysis per serving: *Calories: 238, Fat: 18 g, Saturated Fat: 3 g, Cholesterol: 175 mg, Fiber: 6 g, Protein: 9 g, Carbohydrates: 13 g, Sodium: 578 mg*

AVOCADO, CELERY, AND CITRUS SALAD

Serves: 4

Prep time:
15 minutes

PEGAN DIET

I love the combination of ingredients in this hydrating salad that features a variety of textures, good-quality fats, and a bright citrus blast. This dish is great during the winter, when citrus is in season, but it's equally delicious at the height of summer, when you're craving refreshment. If you want to add a little protein to make this a complete meal, incorporate some thinly sliced grilled chicken breasts.

- 3 tablespoons Homemade Mayonnaise (page 265)
- 1 tablespoon fresh lemon juice
- 1 tablespoon poppy seeds
- ½ teaspoon sea salt
- 2 blood or Valencia oranges
- 1 small head romaine lettuce, torn into bite-size pieces
- 2 avocados, pitted, peeled, and each half cut into 4 slices
- 4 celery ribs, thinly sliced

To make the dressing, in a small bowl, whisk together the mayonnaise, lemon juice, poppy seeds, and salt. If desired, add 1 to 2 tablespoons filtered water to thin the dressing.

Cut off the top and bottom of an orange. Stand the orange on a cut side and, using a sharp knife, cut away the rind and white pith in strips from top to bottom, following the contour of the fruit. Cut the flesh into thin rounds. Repeat with the remaining orange.

Divide the lettuce among 4 plates, then top with the orange rounds, avocado slices, and celery, evenly dividing each ingredient. Using a spoon, drizzle dressing over each salad and serve.

Nutritional analysis per serving: *Calories: 309, Fat: 20 g, Saturated Fat: 2 g, Cholesterol: 5 mg, Fiber: 11 g, Protein: 5 g, Carbohydrates: 31 g, Sodium: 603 mg*

ARTICHOKE, AVOCADO, AND CUCUMBER SALAD

You don't always need lettuce to make a salad. The simple, fresh flavors in this quick-to-prepare dish are a great addition to any lunch or dinner. The salad is also great as a topping for grain-free breads or crackers.

- ¼ cup extra-virgin olive oil
- 2 tablespoons red wine vinegar
- 1 garlic clove, minced
- 2 teaspoons fresh dill, roughly chopped
- ½ teaspoon sea salt
- ¼ teaspoon freshly ground black pepper
- 2 large cucumbers, trimmed
- 1 (14-ounce) can artichoke hearts, rinsed, drained, and roughly chopped
- 1 large avocado, pitted, peeled, and cut into chunks

To make the dressing, in a small bowl, whisk together the olive oil, vinegar, garlic, dill, salt, and pepper.

Slice the cucumbers lengthwise into quarters, then cut each quarter crosswise into ½-inch chunks.

In a large bowl, combine the cucumbers, artichoke hearts, and avocado chunks. Whisk the dressing to recombine. Pour the dressing over the salad and toss well to combine. Let stand for 10 minutes to allow the flavors to mingle. Serve.

Nutritional analysis per serving: *Calories: 528, Fat: 30 g, Saturated Fat: 3 g, Cholesterol: 0 mg, Fiber: 10 g, Protein: 13 g, Carbohydrates: 61 g, Sodium: 958 mg*

HEARTS OF PALM CHOPPED SALAD

Serves: 4

Prep time:
20 minutes

This fantastic recipe with Mexican flair requires very little effort to prepare and absolutely no cooking, but the result is a flavorful, hearty salad. Enhance the dish with some grilled chicken or wild salmon and you will be nourished for hours.

- ¼ cup extra-virgin olive oil
- 2 tablespoons fresh lime juice
- 2 teaspoons fresh oregano leaves, minced
- 1 teaspoon sea salt
- ¼ teaspoon freshly ground black pepper
- ¼ teaspoon crushed red pepper flakes
- 2 large avocados, pitted, peeled, and cut into bite-size chunks
- 1 (14-ounce) can hearts of palm, rinsed, drained, and sliced into ¼-inch-thick rounds
- 1 large red bell pepper, seeded and chopped
- 1¼ cups cherry tomatoes, cut in half
- ½ small red onion, finely diced
- 3 tablespoons toasted unsalted pumpkin seeds
- 2 tablespoons chopped fresh cilantro leaves

To make the dressing, in a jar, combine the olive oil, lime juice, oregano, salt, black pepper, and red pepper flakes. Cover tightly and shake well. The dressing can be refrigerated for up to 2 weeks; bring to room temperature before using.

In a large bowl, combine the avocado, hearts of palm, bell pepper, cherry tomatoes, and red onion. Shake the vinaigrette to recombine, drizzle it over the salad, and toss gently to mix. Sprinkle the salad with the pumpkin seeds and cilantro and serve.

Nutritional analysis per serving: Calories: 297, Fat: 27 g, Saturated Fat: 4 g, Cholesterol: 0 mg, Fiber: 6 g, Protein: 5 g, Carbohydrates: 15 g, Sodium: 804 mg

CAULIFLOWER-HEMP SEED "TABBOULEH"

Serves: 4

Prep time: 30 minutes, plus chilling time

Cauliflower is a fantastic low-carb vegetable that can be transformed to mimic rice and other grains. In this recipe, it replaces the bulgur wheat that's used in traditional tabbouleh.

- 1 head cauliflower, trimmed
- ¼ cup hemp seeds
- 1 bunch parsley, stemmed and roughly chopped
- 2 large tomatoes, cored and diced
- 1 cucumber, diced
- 1 large shallot, minced
- 3 garlic cloves, minced
- ¼ cup extra-virgin olive oil
- grated zest and juice of 1 lemon
- 1 teaspoon sea salt

Using a chef's knife, cut the head of cauliflower in half, then use a paring knife to cut the florets away from the core. Cut the florets into rough 1-inch pieces.

In a food processor, pulse about 2 cups of the florets until broken down into fine bits that resemble grains of rice, 4 or 5 one-second pulses. Transfer to a large bowl and repeat with the remaining cauliflower.

Add the hemp seeds, parsley, tomatoes, cucumber, shallot, garlic, olive oil, lemon zest and juice, and salt to the cauliflower and toss well to combine. Cover and refrigerate for at least 2 hours or up to 3 days. Toss to recombine and serve chilled or at room temperature.

Nutritional analysis per serving: *Calories: 271, Fat: 19 g, Saturated Fat: 2 g, Cholesterol: 0 mg, Fiber: 9 g, Protein: 10 g, Carbohydrates: 24 g, Sodium: 648 mg*

WILD RICE AND WILTED KALE SALAD

PEGAN DIET

Serves: 4

Prep time:
20 minutes,
plus soaking
time

Cook time:
25 minutes,
plus cooling
time

Compared to other whole grains, wild rice is rich in essential minerals. It has a delectable, nutty flavor that pairs perfectly with vegetables of all sorts. This is a super-satisfying salad and a terrific side dish to any type of main dish.

- 1 cup wild rice
- 2 bunches lacinato kale, stemmed and torn into 1-inch pieces
- ¼ cup extra-virgin olive oil
- 1 teaspoon sea salt
- ¼ teaspoon freshly ground black pepper
- 6 large Brussels sprouts, trimmed and shredded
- 1 large carrot, scrubbed and shredded
- ½ red onion, finely chopped
- 2 tablespoons fresh lemon juice
- ¼ cup toasted pumpkin seeds

Put the wild rice in a bowl and cover with 4 cups filtered water. Let soak overnight at room temperature. Drain and rinse well.

Place the rice in a small saucepan and cover with 2½ cups filtered water. Cover, bring to a boil over high heat, then lower the heat to medium and simmer until the rice is tender and has absorbed all the liquid, about 20 minutes. Spread out the rice in a shallow baking dish and allow to cool to room temperature.

Place the kale in a large bowl, drizzle with the olive oil, and sprinkle with the salt and pepper. Using your fingers, gently massage the kale, allowing the leaves to wilt.

Add the cooled wild rice and the Brussels sprouts, carrot, onion, lemon juice, and pumpkin seeds to the kale and toss to combine. Serve.

Nutritional analysis per serving: Calories: 294, Fat: 19 g, Saturated Fat: 3 g, Cholesterol: 0 mg, Fiber: 7 g, Protein: 11 g, Carbohydrates: 26 g, Sodium 633 mg

Quinoa and Black Bean Salad with Mexican Flavors

Serves: 4

Prep time: 20 minutes

Cook time: 20 minutes, plus cooling time

PEGAN DIET

In the last ten years, quinoa has gone from a virtually unknown grain (seeds, to be precise) to a beloved superfood. Naturally gluten-free and loaded with protein, it's a healthy and hearty addition to your diet. This Mexican-inspired salad is great served with grilled chicken or fish.

- 1 cup quinoa, rinsed and drained
- 1 (15-ounce) can black beans, rinsed and drained
- 2 avocados, pitted, peeled, and cut into small chunks
- 1 large red bell pepper, seeded and finely diced
- 1 large tomato, finely diced
- ½ bunch cilantro, roughly chopped
- ¼ cup extra-virgin olive oil
- 2 tablespoons fresh lime juice
- 2 teaspoons ground cumin
- ⅛ teaspoon chipotle powder
- 1 teaspoon sea salt, plus more as needed

Place the quinoa in a saucepan and cover with 2 cups filtered water. Bring to a boil over high heat, then reduce the heat to medium, cover, and simmer until the quinoa is almost tender and has absorbed all the liquid, about 15 minutes. Remove the pan from the heat and let stand, covered, for 5 minutes. Using a fork, fluff the quinoa, spread it out in a shallow baking dish, and allow it to cool to room temperature.

Transfer the cooled quinoa to a large bowl and add the remaining ingredient. Toss until well combined, then taste and adjust the seasoning with more salt, if needed. Serve.

Nutritional analysis per serving: *Calories: 466, Fat: 24 g, Saturated Fat: 3 g, Cholesterol: 0 mg, Fiber: 9 g, Protein: 12 g, Carbohydrates: 54 g, Sodium: 969 mg*

MEDITERRANEAN SARDINE SALAD

Serves: 4

Prep time:
15 minutes

Small oily fish are among the most nutrient-dense foods you can eat. They are also one of the more sustainable options of seafood. Canned sardines are the feature in this simple but delicious salad. For a creamier version, replace the olive oil with an equal amount of Homemade Mayonnaise (page 265).

- 4 (4.37-ounce) cans sardines in water or olive oil, drained
- 2 celery ribs, minced
- 1 small shallot, minced
- 2 garlic cloves, minced
- 6 olive oil–packed sun-dried tomatoes, minced
- 2 large sprigs basil, leaves only, thinly sliced
- 2 tablespoons apple cider vinegar
- ¼ cup extra-virgin olive oil
- ½ teaspoon sea salt
- ½ teaspoon freshly ground black pepper
- 6 cups baby salad greens

Place the sardines in a bowl and use a fork to mash them. Add the celery, shallot, garlic, sun-dried tomatoes, and basil and stir to incorporate. Add the vinegar, olive oil, salt, and pepper and stir until well combined.

Divide the greens among 4 plates. Top each with a portion of the sardine mixture and serve.

Nutritional analysis per serving: *Calories: 353, Fat: 28 g, Saturated Fat: 4 g, Cholesterol: 100 mg, Fiber: 1 g, Protein: 18 g, Carbohydrates: 9 g, Sodium: 568 mg*

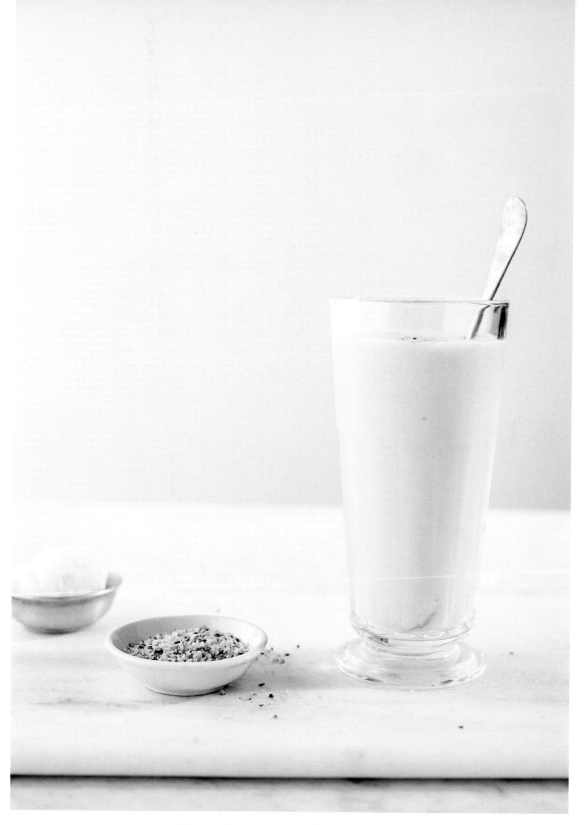

Mango-Coconut Smoothie (page 57)

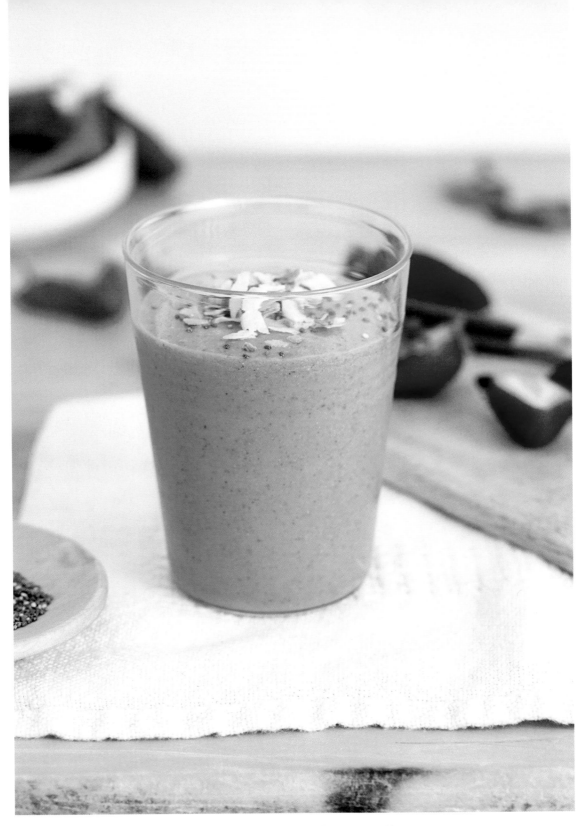

Omega-3 Green Smoothie (page 62)

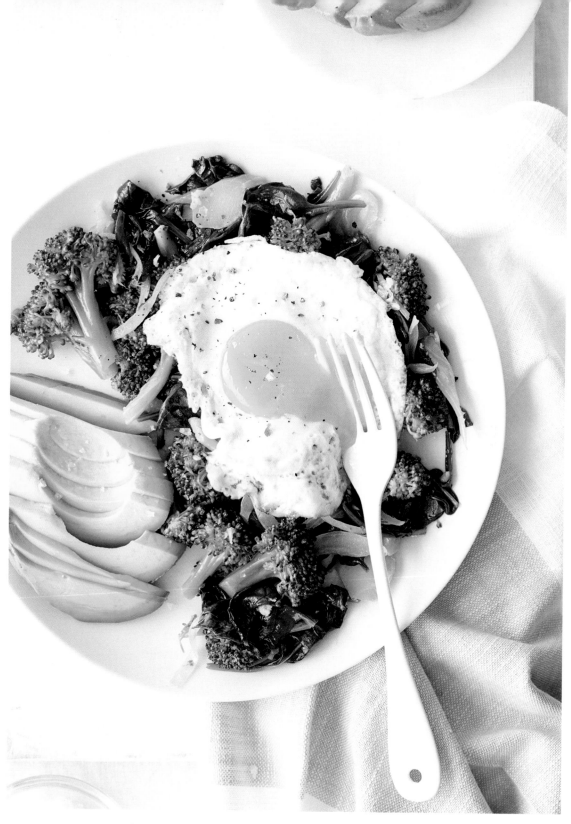

Buttery Broccoli and Spinach with Fried Eggs (page 71)

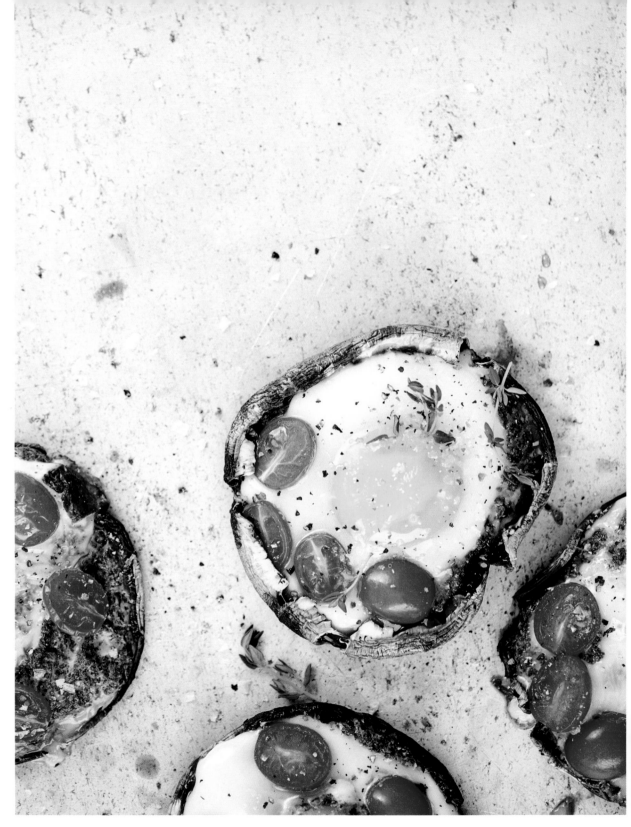

Eggs Baked on Portobello Mushrooms (page 74)

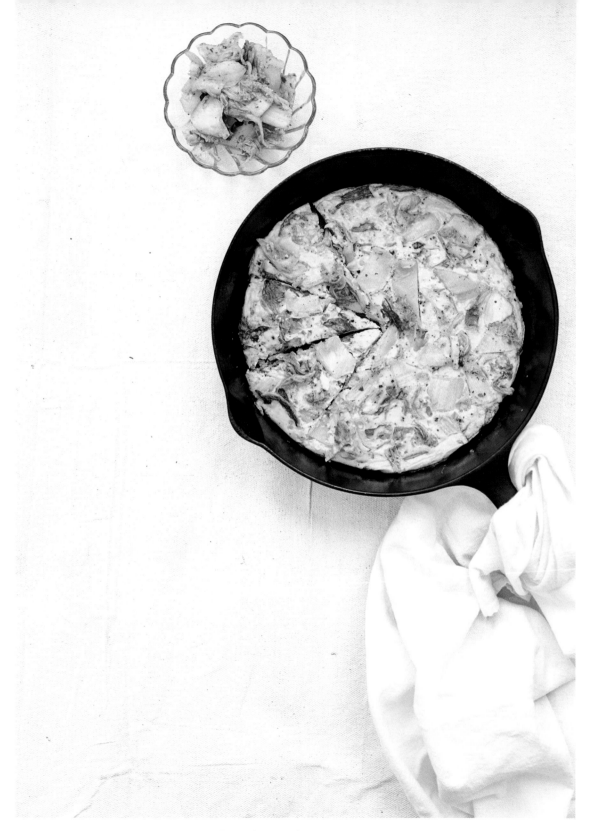

Kimchi and Spinach Frittata (page 79)

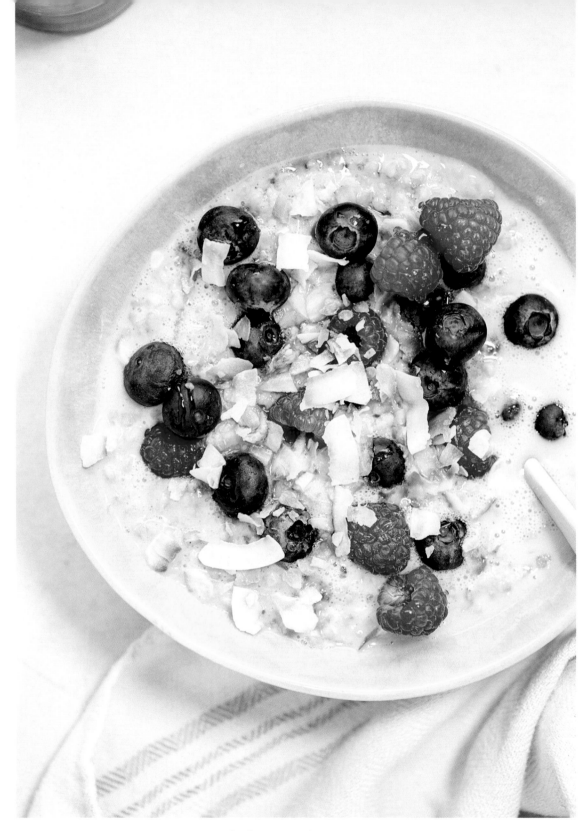

Buckwheat Porridge (page 84)

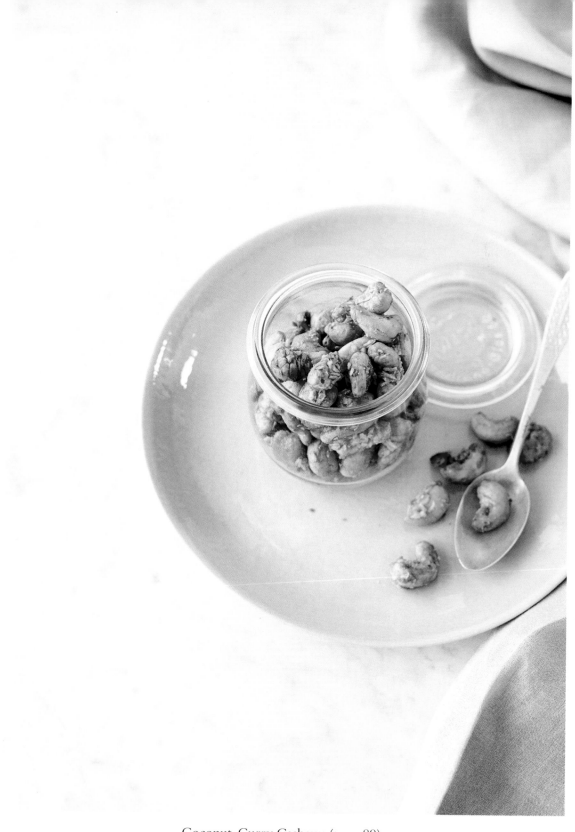

Coconut-Curry Cashews (page 89)

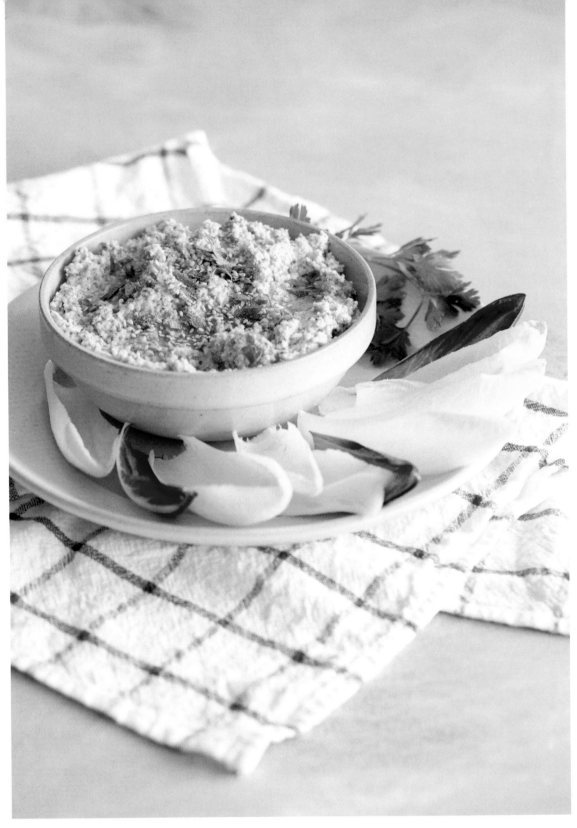

Almond Hummus (page 94)

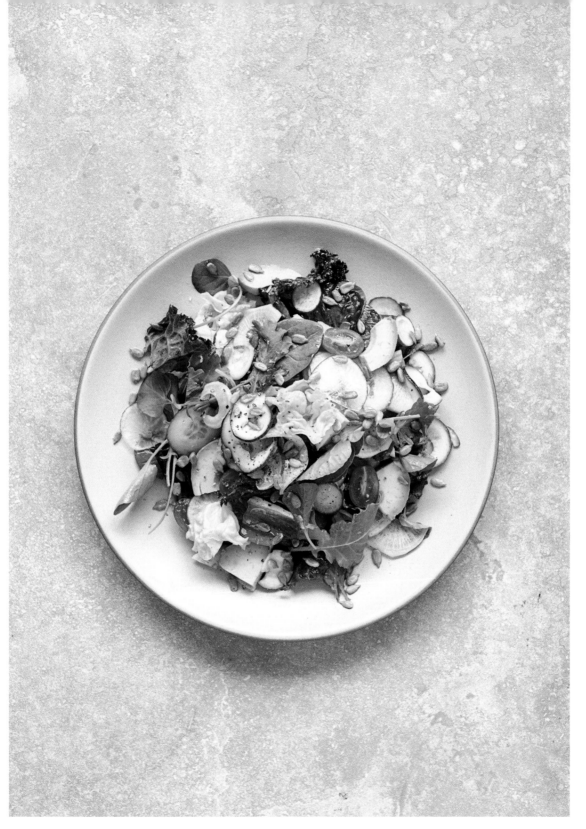

Farmers' Market Salad with Miso Dressing (page 108)

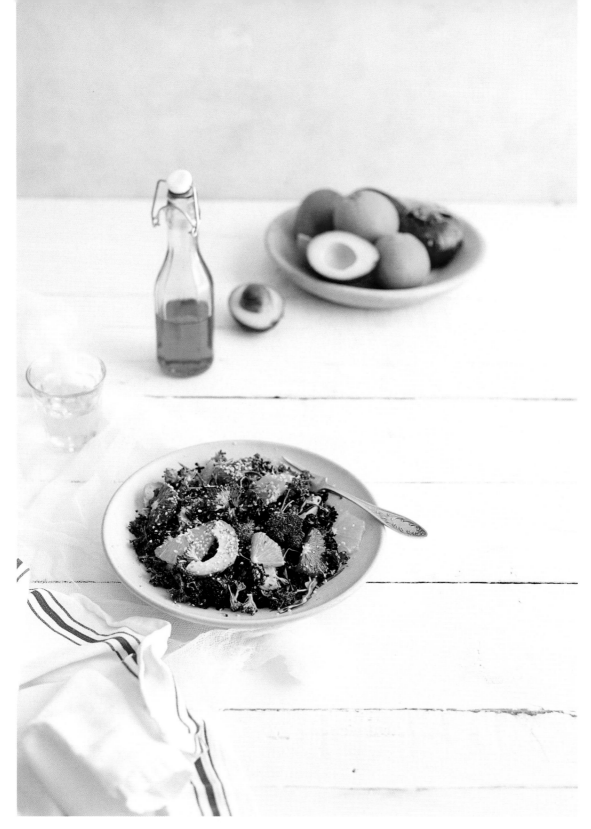

Super Green Salad (page 112)

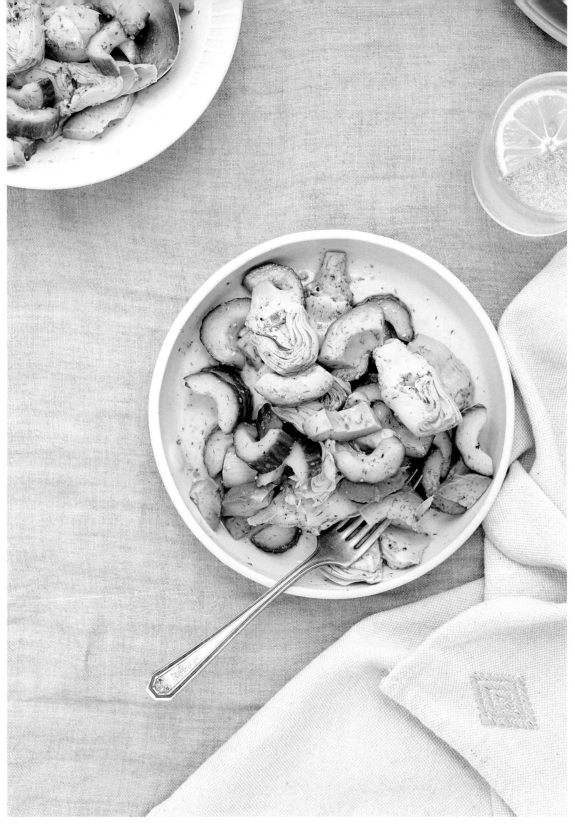

Artichoke, Avocado, and Cucumber Salad (page 115)

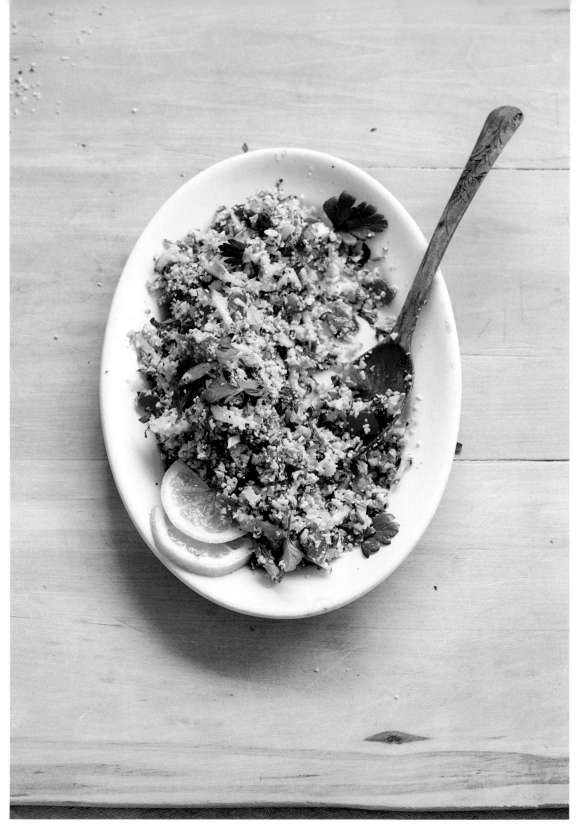

Cauliflower–Hemp Seed "Tabbouleh" (page 117)

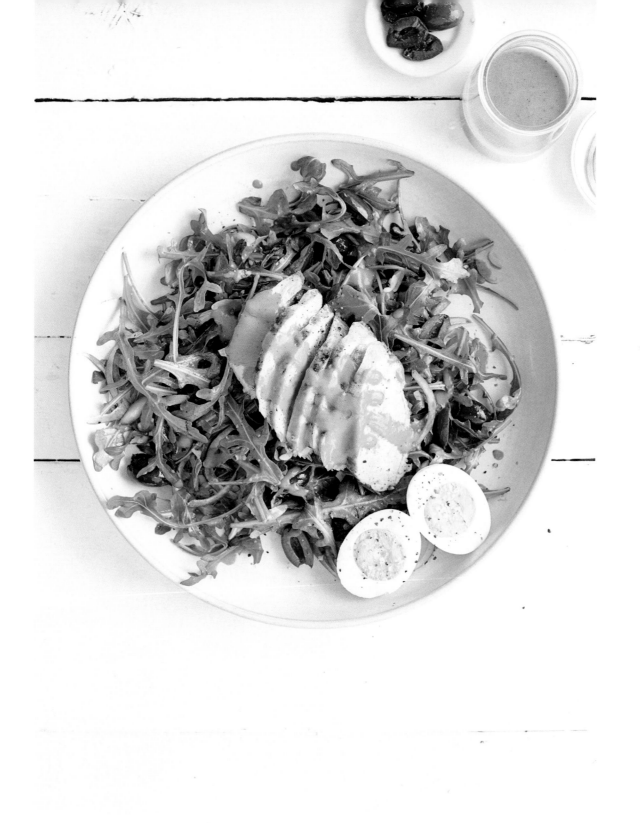

Chicken and Arugula Salad with Roasted Red Pepper Vinaigrette (page 121)

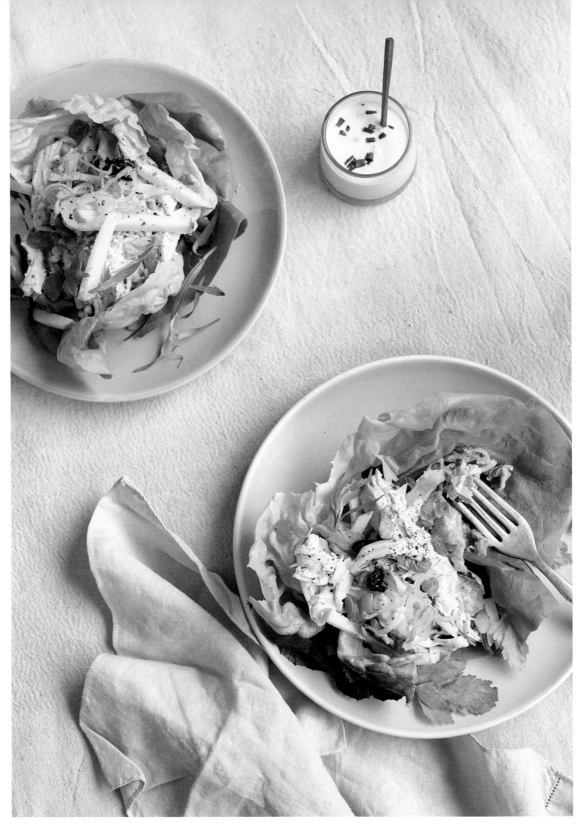

Waldorf Salad with Roasted Chicken (page 123)

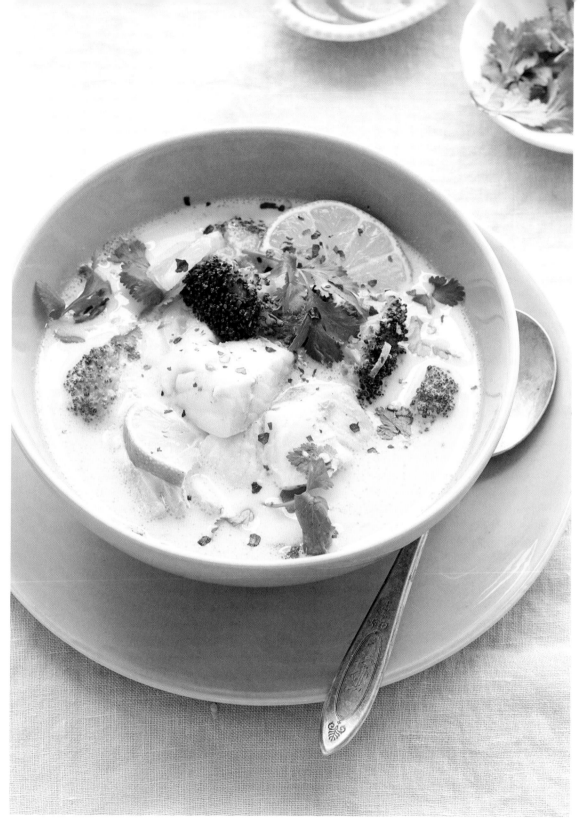

Ginger-Turmeric Fish Soup with Coconut Milk (page 142)

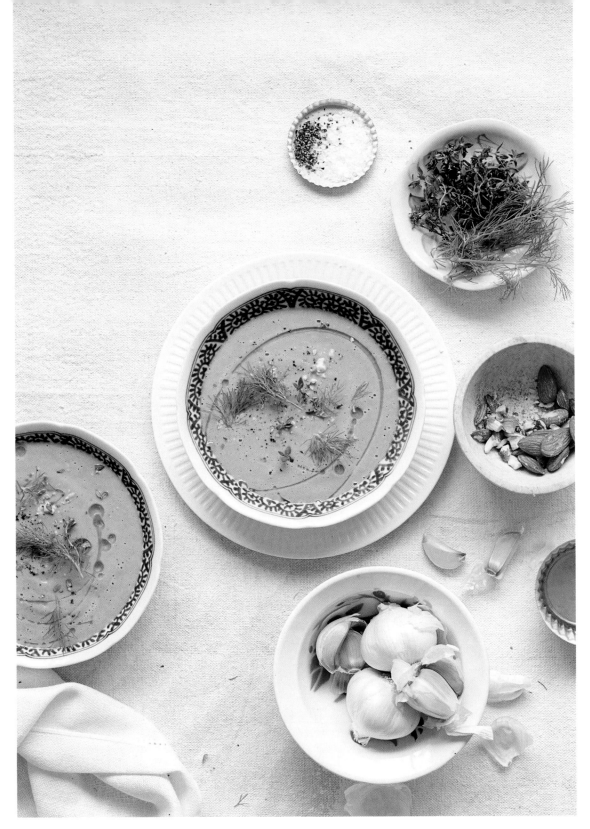

Creamy Fennel and Mushroom Soup (page 146)

CHICKEN AND ARUGULA SALAD WITH ROASTED RED PEPPER VINAIGRETTE

Serves: 4

Prep time: 15 minutes

Cook time: 10 minutes

This is a great main-dish salad that combines high-quality fats from eggs, olives, and extra-virgin olive oil. If you have chicken left over from another meal, use it in place of the chicken breasts and the dish will come together in just a few minutes.

- 4 (6-ounce) boneless, skinless chicken breasts
- ¼ teaspoon freshly ground black pepper
- 1 teaspoon sea salt
- 2 tablespoons avocado oil
- 2 jarred roasted red peppers, patted dry
- ¼ cup extra-virgin olive oil
- 2 tablespoons sherry vinegar
- 2 garlic cloves
- ½ teaspoon dried thyme
- 4 cups baby arugula
- 1 small red onion, thinly sliced
- 1 cup pitted Kalamata olives
- 2 hard-cooked eggs, peeled and quartered

Preheat the oven to 350°F.

Season the chicken breasts on both sides with ½ teaspoon of salt and the pepper.

In a large oven-safe skillet, warm the avocado oil over medium-high heat until shimmering. Add the chicken breasts to the pan in a single layer and cook for 5 minutes. Flip the breasts, transfer the pan to the oven, and cook until the meat is opaque throughout and the internal temperature reaches 165°F on an instant-read thermometer, about 6 to 7 minutes. Transfer the chicken breasts to a cutting board and let rest for 2 to 3 minutes while you make the vinaigrette.

Combine the roasted red peppers, olive oil, vinegar, garlic, thyme, and the remaining salt in a blender. Blend on high speed until smooth, about 30 seconds.

Cut the chicken breasts crosswise into ½-inch slices. Divide the arugula among 4 plates and top with the onion slices, olives, hard-cooked eggs, and chicken, evenly distributing the ingredients. Drizzle vinaigrette over each salad and serve.

Nutritional analysis per serving: *Calories: 507, Fat: 30 g, Saturated Fat: 4 g, Cholesterol: 171 mg, Fiber: 2 g, Protein: 32 g, Carbohydrates: 8 g, Sodium: 1122 mg*

WALDORF SALAD WITH ROASTED CHICKEN

PEGAN DIET

Serves: 4

Prep time:
10 minutes

Cook time:
15 minutes

This classic salad was created at the Waldorf Hotel in the late 1800s and traditionally combines apples, walnuts, celery, and raisins in a creamy dressing. This version includes roasted chicken for protein, and the Homemade Mayo in the dressing adds healthy fats.

- 2 (6-ounce) boneless, skin-on chicken breasts
- ¼ teaspoon freshly ground black pepper
- 2 tablespoons extra-virgin olive oil
- ¾ cup Homemade Mayonnaise (page 265)
- 2 tablespoons apple cider vinegar
- 1 tablespoon Dijon mustard
- 1 tablespoon minced fresh chives
- 1 small shallot, thinly sliced
- 1 Granny Smith apple, cored and cut into ½-inch chunks
- ¾ cup raw walnuts, roughly chopped
- 3 celery ribs, sliced ¼ inch thick
- ¼ cup raisins
- 1 head Bibb lettuce, leaves separated

Preheat the oven to 350°F.

Place the chicken breasts in a small baking dish, season on both sides with the pepper, and drizzle with the olive oil. Turn the breasts skin side down and roast until the meat is opaque throughout and the internal temperature reaches 165°F on an instant-read thermometer, 12 to 15 minutes. Transfer the breasts to a cutting board and allow to cool.

While the chicken cools, in a small bowl, whisk together the mayonnaise, vinegar, mustard, chives, and shallot to make the dressing.

Cut the cooled chicken into ½-inch chunks and place in a large bowl. Add the apple, walnuts, celery, and raisins and the dressing and fold until the mixture is well combined.

Lay the lettuce leaves on 4 plates, dividing them evenly. Scoop the salad mixture onto the lettuce, again dividing evenly, and serve.

Nutritional analysis per serving: Calories: 576, Fat: 38 g, Saturated Fat: 5 g, Cholesterol: 45 mg, Fiber: 0 g, Protein: 14 g, Carbohydrates: 61 g, Sodium: 139 mg

Taco Salad

Serves: 4

Prep time:
30 minutes

Cook time:
10 minutes

Here's a new favorite for Taco Tuesdays! This salad contains all of the spicy flavors of ground beef tacos but isn't weighed down by the heaviness of corn, a common allergen. It's a meal the whole family will love.

- 1 tablespoon coconut oil
- 1 pound grass-fed ground beef
- 2 teaspoons ground cumin
- 1 teaspoon ground coriander
- ¼ teaspoon chipotle powder
- 1 teaspoon dried oregano
- 1 teaspoon sea salt
- 1 avocado, pitted, peeled, and cut into large chunks
- 2 tablespoons extra-virgin olive oil
- ¼ cup fresh cilantro leaves
- 1 garlic clove
- juice of 1 lime
- ¼ teaspoon cayenne pepper
- 7 to 8 cups mesclun
- 2 cups shredded red cabbage
- 2 carrots, scrubbed and shredded
- 1 large tomato, cut into large chunks

In a large skillet, warm the coconut oil over medium-high heat until shimmering. Add the beef and cook, stirring frequently and breaking it into pieces with a wooden spoon, for 2 minutes. Add the cumin, coriander, chipotle powder, oregano, and ½ teaspoon of the salt and continue to cook, stirring occasionally, until the beef is cooked through, about 4 minutes.

Meanwhile, combine the avocado, olive oil, cilantro, garlic, lime juice, cayenne, the remaining ½ teaspoon salt, and ¼ cup filtered water in a blender and blend on high speed until smooth, about 45 seconds. Transfer the dressing to a small serving bowl.

In a large bowl, combine the mesclun, cabbage, carrots, and tomato and toss to combine. Divide the vegetables among 4 plates and top with the beef mixture. Serve, passing the dressing on the side.

Nutritional analysis per serving: Calories: 500, Fat: 31 g, Saturated Fat: 11 g, Cholesterol: 70 mg, Fiber: 17 g, Protein: 28 g, Carbohydrates: 37 g, Sodium: 713 mg

9

Broths and Soups

Dr. Hyman's Veggie-Bone Broth

Makes: 7 to
8 cups

Prep time:
10 minutes

Cook time: 15 to
27 hours
(unattended),
plus cooling
time

Believe the hype! Bone broth is one of the most healing foods you can sip. It's good for your hair, skin, nails, digestion, immune system, and gut. Make bone broth from scratch and be rewarded with a flavorful liquid that supports your entire body.

- 4 pounds beef, lamb, bison, venison, chicken, turkey, and/or duck bones (preferably organic, and grass-fed if using beef)
- 2 tablespoons apple cider vinegar
- 2 carrots, scrubbed and roughly chopped
- 2 celery ribs, roughly chopped
- 1 yellow onion, chopped
- 2 garlic cloves, crushed
- 2 bay leaves
- 1 bunch parsley
- 1 tablespoon sea salt

Place the bones in a 4-quart slow cooker or 4-quart stockpot and drizzle the vinegar over the bones. Add the remaining ingredients to the pot and pour in 2 quarts filtered water. Stir to combine.

If using a slow cooker: cover, set the slow cooker to low, and cook for 12 to 24 hours. If using a stockpot: place the pot on the stove over high heat and bring the water to a boil, then lower the heat to medium and simmer for 8 to 10, and up to as many as 12, hours.

Using a slotted spoon, remove and discard the bones, vegetables, and herbs. Pour the liquid through a fine-mesh sieve into a large glass container and allow to cool. Cover and refrigerate until cold, at least 3 hours.

Using a spoon, skim off and discard the layer of solidified fat on the surface of the broth. Refrigerate the broth in an airtight container for up to 4 days or freeze for up to 1 year.

Nutritional analysis per serving (2 cups): *Calories: 34, Fat: 0 g, Saturated Fat: 0 g, Cholesterol: 0 mg, Fiber: 2 g, Protein: 2 g, Carbohydrates: 8 g, Sodium: 918 mg*

MISO-BUTTER BROTH

Serves: 1

Prep time:
5 minutes

Miso is a Japanese fermented paste traditionally made with soybeans, but there are many soy-free miso options out there, so shop around. Miso-spiked soup boosts the immune system, so sip this broth when you feel sluggish or have a cold coming on.

- 1½ cups Dr. Hyman's Veggie-Bone Broth (page 128), heated
- 1 tablespoon soy-free miso
- 1½ tablespoons unsalted, grass-fed butter

Place all the ingredients in a blender and blend on high speed until well combined, about 30 seconds. Pour the broth into a mug and drink immediately.

Nutritional analysis per serving: Calories: 193, Fat: 17 g, Saturated Fat: 10 g, Cholesterol: 43 mg, Fiber: 0 g, Protein: 1 g, Carbohydrates: 8 g, Sodium: 1514 mg

MINERAL-RICH GREEN SOUP

In the heat of summer, simple raw soups like this are exactly what I crave. The miso in this recipe not only adds delicious flavor; it delivers an array of beneficial bacteria that aid in digestion and help nurture a healthy gut.

- 2 avocados, pitted, peeled, and quartered
- 2 large tomatoes, cored and cut into chunks
- 2 large handfuls baby spinach
- 2 garlic cloves
- 3 scallions, roughly chopped
- 2 tablespoons fresh mint leaves
- 2 tablespoons fresh cilantro leaves
- juice of 1 lemon
- 2 tablespoons soy-free miso
- ¼ cup extra-virgin olive oil
- ¼ teaspoon freshly ground black pepper
- 1½ cups herbal tea (such as holy basil, nettle, or lemon balm), chilled

Combine the avocados, tomatoes, spinach, garlic, scallions, mint, cilantro, lemon juice, miso, oil, and pepper in a blender. Pour in ¾ cup of the herbal tea and blend on high until smooth and creamy, about 30 seconds. Blend in additional tea as needed to thin the soup to the desired consistency. Serve right away or refrigerate in an airtight container for up to 1 day.

Nutritional analysis per serving: *Calories: 487, Fat: 24 g, Saturated Fat: 3 g, Cholesterol: 0 mg, Fiber: 5 g, Protein: 3 g, Carbohydrates: 91 g, Sodium: 262 mg*

CURRIED ZUCCHINI-AVOCADO SOUP

Zucchini is typically paired with Mediterranean flavors, but with a touch of curry powder for spice and avocado for richness, this recipe changes things up a bit. At the height of summer, when the weather is warm, this soup can be enjoyed chilled.

> Serves: 4
>
> Prep time: 10 minutes
>
> Cook time: 10 minutes

- 2 tablespoons Ghee (page 279)
- 2 large zucchini, cut into thin rounds
- 1 large shallot, sliced into thin rounds
- sea salt
- 2 avocados, pitted and peeled; 1 diced for garnish
- 2 tablespoons fresh lime juice
- 2 teaspoons curry powder
- ¼ cup extra-virgin olive oil
- ½ small bunch cilantro, stemmed and roughly chopped

In a saucepan, warm the ghee over medium heat until melted. Add the zucchini and shallot, sprinkle with a little salt, and cook, stirring occasionally, until softened and translucent, 5 to 6 minutes.

Transfer the zucchini mixture to a blender. Add the flesh from 1 avocado to the blender along with the lime juice, curry, and olive oil. Blend on high speed until smooth and creamy, about 45 seconds. If the soup is too thick, add up to ¼ cup filtered water to thin it. Season to taste with salt.

Divide the soup among 4 bowls. Garnish with the cilantro and diced avocado and serve.

Nutritional analysis per serving: *Calories: 336, Fat: 32 g, Saturated Fat: 8 g, Cholesterol: 0 mg, Fiber: 7 g, Protein: 4 g, Carbohydrates: 13 g, Sodium: 584 mg*

Chunky Vegetable and Adzuki Bean Soup with Miso

PEGAN DIET

Serves: 4

Prep time:
30 minutes,
plus soaking
time

Cook time:
1½ hours

Savory miso is known for its immune system–boosting properties. Traditional miso soup was the inspiration for this recipe, but this version is loaded with healthy veggies and protein-rich adzuki beans. Kombu is a wild-harvested seaweed that imparts an earthy flavor and has properties to help cook the beans quicker and make them more digestible.

- 1 cup dried adzuki beans
- 1 small piece kombu
- 1 large leek, white section halved lengthwise, rinsed well, and cut into large chunks
- 8 ounces cremini mushrooms, quartered
- 2 large carrots, scrubbed and cut into ¼-inch-thick rounds
- 1 large turnip, peeled and cut into ½-inch chunks
- 1 (2-inch) piece ginger, peeled and minced
- ½ cup dried wakame (broken into small pieces if in long strands)
- 1 bunch lacinato kale, stemmed and cut into small pieces
- ¼ cup soy-free miso

Put the adzuki beans and kombu in a bowl and cover with 6 cups filtered water. Let soak overnight at room temperature. Drain well.

In a Dutch oven or stockpot, combine the adzuki beans, kombu, leek, mushrooms, carrots, turnip, ginger, and wakame. Pour in 4 cups filtered water and bring to a simmer over medium-high heat. Reduce the heat to medium and cook, stirring occasionally, until the beans are tender, about 1 hour; add more water as needed.

Stir in the kale and cook until the kale is tender, about 15 minutes.

Spoon 1 tablespoon of the miso into each of 4 serving bowls. Ladle about 1½ cups of the soup into each bowl and serve.

Nutritional analysis per serving (1½ cups): *Calories: 355, Fat: 3 g, Saturated Fat: 0 g, Cholesterol: 0 mg, Fiber: 16 g, Protein: 20 g, Carbohydrates: 66 g, Sodium: 1305 mg*

Summer Bounty Vegetable Stew

PEGAN DIET

Serves: 4

Prep time:
20 minutes

Cook time:
45 minutes

Summer vegetables at their peak of freshness, taste, and nutrition are the high-light of this hearty stew. Cumin, chili powder, cilantro, and lime juice lend the dish bold, spicy Mexican flavor accents.

- 2 tablespoons Ghee (page 279)
- 1 large yellow onion, thinly sliced
- 2 celery ribs, sliced ¼ inch thick
- 1 large carrot, scrubbed and cut into ¼-inch-thick rounds
- 2 garlic cloves, minced
- 2 large tomatoes, cored and roughly chopped
- 1 red bell pepper, seeded and thinly sliced
- 2 teaspoons ground cumin
- 1 teaspoon chili powder
- 1 teaspoon dried oregano
- 4 cups Dr. Hyman's Veggie-Bone Broth (page 128)
- 1 zucchini, sliced into ½-inch-thick rounds
- 2 cups of green beans, trimmed and cut into thirds
- 1 (15-ounce) can chickpeas, rinsed and drained
- ¼ cup fresh cilantro leaves, roughly chopped
- juice of 1 lime

In a large saucepan, warm the ghee over medium heat until melted. Add the onion, celery, and carrots and cook, stirring occasionally, until slightly softened, 3 to 4 minutes. Stir in the garlic, tomatoes, bell pepper, cumin, chili powder, and oregano, then pour in the vegetable stock. Bring to a boil, then reduce the heat to medium and simmer until the vegetables are tender, about 15 minutes.

Add the zucchini, green beans, and chickpeas and stir to combine. Continue to simmer until slightly thickened and the zucchini and green beans are tender, 15 to 20 minutes. Stir in the cilantro and lime juice. Serve.

Nutritional analysis per serving: Calories: 374, Fat: 11 g, Saturated Fat: 5 g, Cholesterol: 15 mg, Fiber: 30 g, Protein: 16 g, Carbohydrates: 59 g, Sodium: 518 mg

ROASTED CAULIFLOWER SOUP

This creamy vegan soup features cauliflower, one of my favorite slow carbs. The cauliflower is roasted before simmering to create a really rich flavor that adds lots of depth to this simple soup.

Serves: 4

Prep time: 20 minutes

Cook time: 45 minutes

- 1 large head cauliflower
- 1 large yellow onion, halved, thinly sliced
- ¼ cup extra-virgin olive oil, plus more for drizzling
- 1 teaspoon sea salt, plus more if needed
- ½ teaspoon freshly ground black pepper
- 4 cups unsweetened Almond Milk (page 54)
- 1 bay leaf
- 3 scallions, thinly sliced, green and white parts separated
- ½ cup toasted almonds, roughly chopped

Preheat the oven to 375°F.

Using a chef's knife, cut the head of cauliflower in half, then use a paring knife to cut the florets away from the core. Cut the florets into rough ½-inch pieces.

In a bowl, combine the cauliflower, onion, olive oil, 1 teaspoon of salt, and the pepper. Toss until the vegetables are evenly coated, then distribute in an even layer on a baking sheet. Roast until the cauliflower is golden brown, stirring occasionally, about 20 minutes.

Transfer the cauliflower mixture to a large saucepan and add the almond milk, bay leaf, and white parts of the scallions. Bring to a boil over medium-high heat, then reduce the heat to medium and simmer until the vegetables are completely tender, about 20 minutes.

Discard the bay leaf. Using an immersion blender, puree the mixture directly in the saucepan until mostly smooth but still with some chunks. Taste the soup and adjust the seasoning with more salt, if needed.

Ladle the soup into bowls. Sprinkle with the almonds and the green parts of the scallions, drizzle with olive oil, and serve.

Nutritional analysis per serving: *Calories: 226, Fat: 16 g, Saturated Fat: 2 g, Cholesterol: 0 mg, Fiber: 7 g, Protein: 5 g, Carbohydrates: 17 g, Sodium: 224 mg*

SWEET POTATO SOUP WITH COCONUT AND GINGER

Serves: 4

Prep time:
15 minutes

Cook time:
30 minutes

I love silky, smooth soups like this one. The ginger in this recipe gives the soup a delightful zing and helps offset the sweetness of the sweet potatoes, and the ghee and coconut milk add a richness that will leave you feeling satisfied.

- 2 tablespoons Ghee (page 279)
- 1 large yellow onion, thinly sliced
- 4 garlic cloves, minced
- 1 (2-inch) piece ginger, peeled and minced
- 2 pounds sweet potatoes, peeled and cut into ¼-inch rounds
- 4 cups Dr. Hyman's Veggie-Bone Broth (page 128)
- ½ cup full-fat coconut milk
- 1 teaspoon sea salt
- 4 scallions, thinly sliced
- 4 tablespoons unsalted, grass-fed butter

In a 4-quart saucepan, warm the ghee over medium heat until melted. Add the onion and cook, stirring occasionally, until softened and translucent, 3 to 4 minutes. Stir in the garlic and ginger and cook until fragrant, about 2 minutes. Add the sweet potatoes, stir to incorporate, and pour in the bone broth. Bring the liquid to a simmer, cover, and cook until the sweet potatoes are tender, about 20 minutes.

Carefully transfer the contents of the pot to a blender. Pour in the coconut milk and blend on high speed until smooth and creamy, about 45 seconds. Do not fill the blender more than halfway, as hot liquids expand when blending. Keep the lid on tight and cover with a folded kitchen towel, holding the lid down as you blend. Start the speed on low and gradually increase to high speed.

Return the soup to the saucepan and warm over medium heat. Stir in the salt and scallions and ladle the soup into 4 bowls. Top each portion with 1 tablespoon of the butter and serve.

Nutritional analysis per serving: *Calories: 520, Fat: 23 g, Saturated Fat: 14 g, Cholesterol: 35 mg, Fiber: 8 g, Protein: 9 g, Carbohydrates: 58 g, Sodium: 744 mg*

CREAMY POTATO SOUP WITH DULSE FLAKES

Serves: 4

Prep time:
15 minutes

Cook time:
45 minutes

PEGAN DIET

Dulse is a wild seaweed loaded with vitamins and minerals, including B$_6$, B$_{12}$, iron, and potassium. It has a unique flavor that adds a delicious, savory character to this creamy soup. You can find dried dulse flakes in most health-food stores.

- 2 tablespoons Ghee (page 279)
- 1 large onion, thinly sliced
- 3 celery ribs, sliced ¼ inch thick
- 3 garlic cloves, minced
- 2½ pounds Yukon Gold potatoes, peeled, cut into quarters
- 4 cups chicken or vegetable stock
- 1 tablespoon dried thyme
- 1 teaspoon ground fennel seeds
- 1 bay leaf
- 4 tablespoons unsalted, grass-fed butter
- 2 tablespoons dulse flakes
- ½ teaspoon freshly ground white pepper

In a large saucepan, warm the ghee over medium-high heat until melted. Add the onion and celery and cook, stirring occasionally, until the vegetables are slightly softened, 3 to 4 minutes. Stir in the garlic and cook until fragrant, about 1 minute. Add the potatoes, stock, thyme, fennel seeds, and bay leaf. Bring to a boil, reduce the heat to medium, and simmer uncovered, stirring occasionally, until the potatoes are very tender, about 30 minutes.

Remove and discard the bay leaf. Place about half the soup mixture in a blender along with 2 tablespoons of the butter and blend on high speed until creamy. Do not fill the blender more than halfway, as hot liquids expand when blending. Keep the lid on tight and cover with a folded kitchen towel, holding the lid down as you blend. Start the speed on low and gradually increase to high speed. Transfer to a bowl and repeat with the remaining soup mixture and the remaining butter.

Return the pureed soup to the saucepan and warm over medium heat, stirring occasionally, until hot throughout. Stir in the dulse flakes and white pepper and serve.

Nutritional analysis per serving: Calories: 402, Fat: 12 g, Saturated Fat: 6 g, Cholesterol: 11 mg, Fiber: 6 g, Protein: 13 g, Carbohydrates: 63 g, Sodium: 410 mg

RICH ONION SOUP

Onions contain powerful phytochemicals that can help reduce inflammation. This onion soup, a favorite of mine in the winter months, also provides immune support because it's made with bone broth.

- 1 tablespoon Ghee (page 279)
- 2½ pounds yellow onions, thinly sliced
- 1 cup dry white wine
- 2 bay leaves
- 3 garlic cloves, minced
- 1 (2- by 6-inch) piece kombu
- 1 tablespoon dried thyme
- 2 teaspoons dried oregano
- 8 cups Dr. Hyman's Veggie-Bone Broth (page 128)
- 2 tablespoons wheat-free tamari
- 6 tablespoons unsalted, grass-fed butter, at room temperature
- ½ bunch parsley, stemmed and roughly chopped

Serves: 4

Prep time: 15 minutes

Cook time: 1 hour

In a large pot, warm the ghee over medium-high heat until melted. Add the onions and cook, stirring occasionally, until softened and golden brown, 15 to 20 minutes; reduce the heat to medium if the onions are browning too quickly. Pour in the wine and add the bay leaves, garlic, kombu, thyme, and oregano. Simmer until the wine has reduced by half, then pour in the bone broth. Bring to a simmer, reduce the heat to maintain a gentle simmer, and cook, partially covered, for 45 minutes.

Stir the tamari into the soup. Remove and discard the bay leaves and kombu and ladle the soup into 4 serving bowls. Top each portion with 1½ tablespoons of the butter, sprinkle with parsley, and serve.

Nutritional analysis per serving: *Calories: 621, Fat: 27 g, Saturated Fat: 14 g, Cholesterol: 56 mg, Fiber: 24 g, Protein: 28 g, Carbohydrates: 66 g, Sodium: 755 mg*

Hearty Lentil and Mushroom Soup

Serves: 4

Prep time:
20 minutes,
plus soaking
time

Cook time:
1¾ hours

PEGAN DIET

This is a classic lentil soup with a twist: Cremini mushrooms make the protein-rich soup even heartier and give it a deep, meaty flavor. Leftovers keep well, so make a double batch and enjoy the soup over the week.

- 1½ cups green lentils
- 2 tablespoons Ghee (page 279)
- 1 large yellow onion, roughly chopped
- 4 cups thinly sliced cremini mushrooms
- 3 celery ribs, cut into ½-inch pieces
- 2 large carrots, scrubbed and cut into ¼-inch rounds
- 4 cups Dr. Hyman's Veggie-Bone Broth (page 128) or filtered water
- ¼ cup dulse flakes
- 2 bay leaves
- 2 teaspoons garlic powder
- 1 (6-inch) sprig rosemary, leaves only, finely chopped
- 1 teaspoon dried basil
- ½ teaspoon freshly ground black pepper
- ½ bunch parsley, stemmed and roughly chopped

Put the lentils in a bowl and cover with 4 cups filtered water. Let soak overnight at room temperature.

Drain the lentils in a colander and set aside.

In a 4-quart saucepan, warm the ghee over medium–high heat until melted. Add the onion and mushrooms and cook, stirring occasionally, until softened, 3 to 4 minutes. Stir in the celery, carrots, and lentils and cook until heated through. Add the bone broth, dulse flakes, bay leaves, garlic powder, rosemary, and basil and stir to combine. Cover and bring to a boil, then reduce the heat to medium and simmer until the lentils and vegetables are completely tender, about 1½ hours.

Season the soup with the pepper to taste. Stir in the parsley and serve.

Nutritional analysis per serving: *Calories: 234, Fat: 8 g, Saturated Fat: 5 g, Cholesterol: 2 mg, Fiber: 11 g, Protein: 12 g, Carbohydrates: 30 g, Sodium: 2968 mg*

Ginger-Turmeric Fish Soup with Coconut Milk

Serves: 4

Prep time:
20 minutes

Cook time:
30 minutes

Ginger and turmeric are ingredients with anti–inflammatory properties, and both infuse this soup with exotic fragrance and flavor. For best taste and texture, I recommend using at least two different kinds of whitefish, but the soup will still be delicious if made with only one type.

- 1 tablespoon Ghee (page 279)
- 1 small yellow onion, thinly sliced
- 1 tablespoon peeled and minced ginger
- 1 tablespoon peeled and minced fresh turmeric or 1 teaspoon ground turmeric
- 2 garlic cloves, minced
- 1 (13.5-ounce) can full-fat coconut milk
- 2 cups chicken stock
- 2 tablespoons fish sauce
- 1 tablespoon rice vinegar
- 1 large broccoli crown, stems peeled and finely diced, florets cut into 1-inch pieces
- 1 pound skinless whitefish fillets (such as cod, halibut, haddock, striped bass), cut into 1-inch chunks
- ½ cup loosely packed fresh cilantro leaves, roughly chopped
- crushed red pepper, for garnish (optional)
- 1 lime, cut into 8 wedges

In a Dutch oven, warm the ghee over medium heat until melted. Add the onion and cook, stirring occasionally, until softened and translucent, 3 to 4 minutes. Stir in the ginger, turmeric, and garlic and cook until fragrant, about 1 minute. Add the coconut milk, chicken stock, fish sauce, and vinegar, bring to a simmer, and cook for 10 minutes. Stir in the broccoli and cook until tender, about 5 minutes. Add the fish, gently stir, and cook until the fish is opaque throughout, about 5 minutes. Gently stir in the cilantro.

Ladle the soup into bowls, garnish with crushed red pepper, if using, and serve with the lime wedges on the side.

Nutritional analysis per serving: Calories: 314, Fat: 15 g, Saturated Fat: 10 g, Cholesterol: 54 mg, Fiber: 4 g, Protein: 27 g, Carbohydrates: 19 g, Sodium: 1016 mg

Chicken, Vegetable, and Lentil Soup

Serves: 4

Prep time:
30 minutes

Cook time:
1 hour

PEGAN DIET

This is comfort food at its best. Nutritious veggies combined with healing bone broth, protein-dense lentils, and chicken yield a soup that's a complete lunch or dinner in a bowl.

- 2 tablespoons coconut oil
- 1 large yellow onion, thinly sliced
- 2 celery ribs, sliced ¼ inch thick
- 2 small carrots, scrubbed and cut into ¼-inch rounds
- 2 garlic cloves, minced
- 1 tablespoon tomato paste
- 2 large boneless, skinless chicken breasts, sliced crosswise into ¼-inch strips
- 1 tablespoon dried oregano
- 1 cup green lentils, rinsed
- 5 cups Dr. Hyman's Veggie-Bone Broth (page 128)
- 1 small head cauliflower, trimmed
- 1 tablespoon sea salt
- ½ cup toasted almonds, coarsely chopped

In a Dutch oven, warm the coconut oil over medium heat until melted. Add the onion, celery, and carrots and cook, stirring occasionally, until the vegetables have softened, 4 to 5 minutes. Stir in the garlic and tomato paste and cook until fragrant and well combined, 2 to 3 minutes. Add the chicken, oregano, lentils, and stock and stir to combine. Bring to a simmer, then reduce heat to medium-low, cover, and cook for 30 minutes, stirring occasionally, until the lentils are just shy of tender.

While the soup is simmering, using a paring knife, cut the cauliflower florets away from the core; discard the core. Cut the florets into 1-inch pieces.

Add the cauliflower to the pot, stir to combine, and continue to cook, covered, until the cauliflower and lentils are tender, about 15 minutes.

Stir in the salt and serve, sprinkling each portion with about 2 tablespoons of the chopped almonds.

Nutritional analysis per serving: *Calories: 685, Fat: 34 g, Saturated Fat: 11 g, Cholesterol: 42 mg, Fiber: 41 g, Protein: 35 g, Carbohydrates: 80 g, Sodium: 734 mg*

CREAMY FENNEL AND MUSHROOM SOUP

Serves: 4

Prep time:
20 minutes

Cook time:
40 minutes

Fennel, traditionally used in Mediterranean cuisine, is a flavorful plant that has a sort of licorice taste. Ancient medicine uses fennel for an assortment of ailments, including an upset stomach and congestion. Blended with healing mushrooms, this soup will warm you up on a cold day or help soothe any symptoms of a cold.

- 1 large leek
- 1 large fennel bulb
- 5 large portobello mushrooms
- 1 tablespoon Ghee (page 279)
- 1 teaspoon sea salt
- 3 garlic cloves, minced
- 1 cup dry white wine
- 3 cups unsweetened almond milk
- 1 large sprig thyme, leaves only, well chopped (about 1 teaspoon)
- ¼ teaspoon freshly ground black pepper
- 1 tablespoon extra-virgin olive oil

Remove the leek top. Cut away the root, then slice the white section in half lengthwise and rinse under running water to remove any dirt that may have accumulated. Cut the leek halves into ½-inch pieces and set aside.

Trim off the fennel fronds and reserve for the garnish, then cut the bulb into quarters. Cut away the core, then slice the bulb into thin strips and set aside.

Remove the stems from the mushrooms and then use a spoon to carefully scrape away the gills, which are often full of dirt. Cut the mushrooms into ¼-inch-thick strips.

Add the ghee to a large stockpot and heat over medium heat until melted. Add the leeks and cook for 2 to 3 minutes, stirring occasionally. Stir in the fennel and continue cooking for another 2 to 3 minutes. Add the mushrooms, sprinkle in ½ teaspoon of the salt to help release their juices, and cook for 3 to 4 minutes, stirring occasionally and allowing them to brown slightly.

Stir in the garlic, cook until fragrant (about 45 seconds), then pour in the white wine. Turn up the heat to medium–high and allow the wine to reduce by half. Pour in 2 cups of the almond milk, lower the heat back to medium, and simmer for 20 minutes.

Remove the pot from the heat and pour the contents into a blender. Do not fill the blender more than halfway, as hot liquids expand when blending. Keep the lid on tight and cover with a folded kitchen towel, holding the lid down as you blend. Start the speed on low and gradually increase to high speed. Slowly add the remaining almond milk as you are blending, to thin the soup.

Pour the soup back into the pan and cook over low heat for 2 minutes. Stir in the thyme and season the soup with the remaining salt and the pepper.

Serve the soup garnished with a few chopped fennel fronds and topped with a little drizzle of the olive oil.

Nutritional analysis per serving: *Calories: 223, Fat: 9 g, Saturated Fat: 3 g, Cholesterol: 0 mg, Fiber: 5 g, Protein: 21 g, Carbohydrates: 14 g, Sodium: 612 mg*

10

Vegetables (Side Dishes and Main Dishes)

SAVORY COCONUT PANCAKES

Makes:
12 (1-inch)
pancakes

Prep time:
10 minutes

Cook time:
10 minutes

These lightly spicy pancakes are quick and easy to make. Serve them topped with Shredded Chicken (page 201), with a savory cashew cream, or simply with grass-fed butter.

- 4 large eggs
- ¼ cup coconut flour
- 1 teaspoon sea salt
- 1 teaspoon baking powder
- 1 teaspoon ground cumin
- 2 tablespoons roughly chopped fresh cilantro
- ¼ teaspoon chipotle powder
- Ghee (page 279), for greasing the pan

Crack the eggs into a large bowl and whisk gently. Add the coconut flour, salt, baking powder, cumin, cilantro, chipotle powder, and 2 tablespoons filtered water and whisk to combine. Let the batter stand for 5 minutes.

In an 8-inch skillet, warm 1 tablespoon ghee over medium heat until melted. Pour 2-tablespoon amounts of batter into the skillet, forming as many pancakes as will comfortably fit, and cook for 2 minutes. Use a metal spatula to flip each pancake, and continue to cook until the pancakes are slightly firm to the touch, about 1 more minute. Transfer the pancakes to a large plate. Grease the skillet with more ghee and repeat with the remaining batter.

Serve the pancakes warm or at room temperature.

Nutritional analysis per serving (3 pancakes): *Calories: 240, Fat: 21 g, Saturated Fat: 12 g, Cholesterol: 185 mg, Fiber: 3 g, Protein: 7 g, Carbohydrates: 5 g, Sodium: 523 mg*

White Bean Puree with Rosemary

Makes: 2 cups

Prep time:
15 minutes, plus
soaking time

Cook time:
30 minutes

PEGAN DIET

Silky smooth and seasoned with fresh rosemary, this simple bean puree is a great side dish to roasted vegetables and grilled chicken, lamb, or beef. Although they may not agree with everyone, white beans contain essential nutrients and fiber that can improve cholesterol profiles. So feel free to try this puree after completing the twenty-one-day plan.

- 1 cup dried cannellini beans
- 1 tablespoon apple cider vinegar
- 1 tablespoon Ghee (page 279)
- 1 small onion, thinly sliced
- 3 garlic cloves, minced
- 2½ cups chicken stock
- 1 bay leaf
- 2 tablespoons unsalted, grass-fed butter
- 1 (4-inch) sprig rosemary, leaves only, finely chopped
- 1 teaspoon sea salt
- ½ teaspoon freshly ground black pepper

Put the cannellini beans in a bowl, add the vinegar, and cover with 4 cups warm filtered water. Let soak at room temperature for at least 8 hours or up to 12 hours.

Drain the beans in a colander, rinse well, and set aside.

In a large saucepan, warm the ghee over medium heat until melted. Add the onion and cook, stirring occasionally, until softened and translucent, 3 to 4 minutes. Stir in the garlic and cook until fragrant, about 1 minute, then add the beans, 2 cups of the chicken stock, and the bay leaf. Bring to a simmer, cover partially, and simmer until the beans are very tender, 20 to 25 minutes.

Remove and discard the bay leaf. Transfer the beans and their cooking liquid to a blender, pour in the remaining chicken stock, and add the butter. Do not fill the blender more than halfway, as hot liquids expand when blending. Keep the lid on tight and cover with a folded kitchen towel, holding the lid down as you blend. Start the speed on low and gradually increase to high speed. Blend until smooth and creamy, about 45 seconds.

Return the puree to the saucepan and stir in the rosemary, salt, and pepper. Warm over low heat, stirring occasionally, until heated through. Serve.

Nutritional analysis per serving (½ cup): *Calories: 279, Fat: 11 g, Saturated Fat: 6 g, Cholesterol: 71 mg, Fiber: 10 g, Protein: 12 g, Carbohydrates: 1 g, Sodium: 788 mg*

ITALIAN MARINATED VEGETABLES

Serves: 4

Prep time:
20 minutes,
plus chilling
time

This recipe features an assortment of delicious veggies and is a perfect side dish to just about any meal. Marinated veggies are also great for snacking on throughout the day. Eat the rainbow!

- 2 large carrots, scrubbed and trimmed
- 1 large fennel bulb, trimmed
- 1 small shallot, peeled
- 1 large broccoli crown, stems peeled and cut into ¼-inch rounds, florets cut into 1-inch pieces
- 2 tablespoons extra-virgin olive oil
- ¼ cup apple cider vinegar
- ¼ cup fresh lemon juice
- ¼ cup dulse flakes
- ½ tablespoon Dijon mustard
- 1 tablespoon nutritional yeast
- 1 teaspoon dried thyme
- 1 teaspoon dried oregano
- 1 teaspoon onion powder
- ½ teaspoon garlic powder
- ¼ teaspoon freshly ground black pepper

Use a mandolin or a sharp chef's knife to slice the carrots into ⅛-inch coins. Slice the fennel across the grain into ⅛-inch pieces, then slice the shallot into ⅛-inch rounds. Place the sliced vegetables in a large bowl along with the broccoli.

In a separate bowl, whisk together the remaining ingredients until well combined.

Pour the dressing over the vegetables and toss gently until evenly coated. Cover and refrigerate for at least 20 minutes or up to 8 hours. Serve chilled.

Nutritional analysis per serving: *Calories: 256, Fat: 21 g, Saturated Fat: 3 g, Cholesterol: 0 mg, Fiber: 7 g, Protein: 5 g, Carbohydrates: 15 g, Sodium: 175 mg*

CONFETTI VEGETABLE SLAW WITH TAHINI DRESSING

Serves: 4

Prep time:
20 minutes

Tahini is filled with vitamins and minerals that promote healthy cell growth, and it's also a great source of protein and healthy fat. Here, tahini is mixed with phytonutrient-rich veggies to make a side dish that is the perfect accompaniment to any main course.

- 1 large carrot, scrubbed
- 2 large beets, peeled
- 1 large watermelon radish, peeled
- 1 turnip, peeled
- ½ cup unsalted tahini
- ¼ cup fresh lemon juice
- 3 garlic cloves
- 1 teaspoon sea salt
- ½ cup packed fresh parsley leaves, roughly chopped
- 2 scallions, thinly sliced
- ¼ cup toasted unsalted pumpkin seeds

Using the large holes of a box grater or a food processor fitted with the medium shredding disk, grate the carrot, beets, radish, and turnip. As they are grated, place the vegetables in a large bowl.

Combine the tahini, lemon juice, garlic, salt, and 1 cup filtered water in a blender. Blend on high speed until well combined, then transfer to a small bowl. Stir in the parsley and scallions.

Pour the dressing over the vegetables and stir until evenly coated. Sprinkle with the pumpkin seeds and serve.

Nutritional analysis per serving: *Calories: 275, Fat: 20 g, Saturated Fat: 5 g, Cholesterol: 0 mg, Fiber: 7 g, Protein: 9 g, Carbohydrates: 19 g, Sodium: 686 mg*

RED CABBAGE SLAW WITH CUMIN

Serves: 4

Prep time:
15 minutes,
plus marinating
time

Everyone needs a go-to recipe for slaw, and this cumin-spiked version is the one I always turn to. It's especially good with grilled chicken or fish.

- 1 small head red cabbage, finely shredded
- 2 red bell peppers, seeded and sliced into thin strips
- 1 large carrot, scrubbed and grated
- 2 large tomatoes, cored and finely diced
- 1 bunch parsley, stemmed and roughly chopped
- 1 tablespoon cumin seed
- ¼ cup extra-virgin olive oil
- 1½ tablespoons apple cider vinegar
- 1 teaspoon sea salt

In a large bowl, combine all the ingredients and toss well. Let stand for 10 to 15 minutes at room temperature to allow the flavors to mingle. Serve.

Nutritional analysis per serving: Calories: 220, Fat: 14 g, Saturated Fat: 2 g, Cholesterol: 0 mg, Fiber: 6 g, Protein: 4 g, Carbohydrates: 22 g, Sodium: 514 mg

GINGER-TURMERIC CABBAGE

Serves: 4

Prep time:
5 minutes

Cook time:
10 minutes

Turmeric is a healing spice known for its anti–inflammatory properties. I make sure to use it whenever I have a cold or feel that my immune system needs a boost. Pair this dish with a side of bone broth for an extra-healing meal.

- 2 tablespoons Ghee (page 279) or avocado oil
- 1 small head napa cabbage, shredded
- 1 (2-inch) piece ginger, peeled and grated
- ½ teaspoon ground turmeric
- ¼ teaspoon freshly ground black pepper
- 1 tablespoon low-sodium, wheat-free tamari
- 1 tablespoon rice vinegar

In a 10-inch skillet, warm the ghee over medium–high heat until shimmering. Add the cabbage and cook, tossing continuously, until wilted and the volume has reduced by about half, 2 to 3 minutes. Add the ginger, turmeric, and pepper and stir to combine. Drizzle in the tamari and vinegar, toss to incorporate, and serve.

Nutritional analysis per serving: *Calories: 138, Fat: 10 g, Saturated Fat: 5 g, Cholesterol: 0 mg, Fiber: 0 g, Protein: 5 g, Carbohydrates: 11 g, Sodium: 276 mg*

Cauliflower "Rice" with Scallions

Serves: 4

Prep time:
5 minutes

Cook time:
10 minutes

You won't miss regular rice with this veggie alternative. Cauliflower "rice" will quickly become a staple recipe in your collection. It's easy to prepare and cooks more quickly than actual rice.

- 1 head cauliflower, trimmed
- 2 tablespoons extra-virgin olive oil
- 1 teaspoon sea salt
- 3 scallions, thinly sliced

Using a chef's knife, cut the head of cauliflower in half, then use a paring knife to cut the florets away from the core. Cut the florets and the core into rough ½-inch pieces.

In a food processor, pulse about 2 cups of the cauliflower pieces until broken down into fine bits that resemble grains of rice, 6 to 8 two-second pulses. Transfer to a large bowl and repeat with the remaining cauliflower.

In a 10-inch skillet, warm the olive oil over medium heat until shimmering. Add the cauliflower and cook, stirring frequently, until tender, 4 to 5 minutes. Stir in the salt and scallions and serve.

Nutritional analysis per serving: *Calories: 92, Fat: 7 g, Saturated Fat: 1 g, Cholesterol: 0 mg, Fiber: 3 g, Protein: 3 g, Carbohydrates: 7 g, Sodium: 478 mg*

CURRIED CAULIFLOWER WITH PEAS AND MINT

Serves: 4

Prep time:
10 minutes

Cook time:
15 minutes

This flavorful curried cauliflower dish is the perfect accompaniment to slow-cooked lamb, grilled chicken, or even grilled tofu.

- 1 large head cauliflower, trimmed
- 2 tablespoons Ghee (page 279)
- 1 small red onion, thinly sliced
- 1 tablespoon curry powder
- 1 teaspoon sea salt
- ¼ cup chicken or vegetable stock
- 1 cup fresh or defrosted frozen peas
- ¼ cup dried currants
- ¼ cup unsalted roasted cashews
- 2 tablespoons julienned fresh mint leaves
- juice of 1 lemon

Using a paring knife, cut the cauliflower florets away from the core; discard the core. Cut the florets into 1-inch pieces.

In a large skillet over medium-high heat, warm the ghee until melted. Add the onion and cook, stirring occasionally, until softened, 2 to 3 minutes. Add the cauliflower, curry powder, and salt, toss to combine, and cook for 2 minutes. Pour in the stock, cover, and cook until the cauliflower is tender, 3 to 4 minutes.

Add the peas to the cauliflower and stir to combine. Fold in the currants, cashews, mint, and lemon juice and serve.

Nutritional analysis per serving: *Calories: 213, Fat: 12 g, Saturated Fat: 5 g, Cholesterol: 0 mg, Fiber: 6 g, Protein: 7 g, Carbohydrates: 24 g, Sodium: 697 mg*

Asparagus with Toasted Hazelnuts and Lemon

Asparagus is packed with glutathione, the mother of all antioxidants and a powerful detoxifier that has been shown to help prevent aging, cancer, heart disease, and dementia. Serve this side dish alongside roasted fish, grilled tofu, or seared steak.

- 1 teaspoon sea salt
- 2 pounds asparagus, trimmed
- 2 tablespoons unsalted, grass-fed butter
- ½ cup hazelnuts, coarsely chopped
- 1 large shallot, sliced into ¼-inch rounds
- grated zest and juice of 1 lemon
- ¼ teaspoon freshly ground black pepper

In a Dutch oven or stockpot, bring 6 cups filtered water to a simmer over medium-high heat. Meanwhile, fill a large bowl with ice water.

Add ½ teaspoon of the salt and the asparagus to the simmering water and cook until the asparagus is tender, 3 to 4 minutes. Drain immediately and transfer the asparagus to the ice water to stop the cooking. Once the asparagus has chilled, drain again and set aside.

In a large sauté pan, warm the butter over medium heat until melted. Add the hazelnuts and shallot and cook, stirring occasionally, until the shallots soften and the hazelnuts are golden brown, about 3 minutes. Add the asparagus and toss to combine. Sprinkle in the lemon zest and juice along with the remaining salt and pepper. Toss again to combine and cook just until the asparagus is heated through, 30 to 60 seconds. Transfer to a platter and serve.

Nutritional analysis per serving: *Calories: 186, Fat: 15 g, Saturated Fat: 4 g, Cholesterol: 15 mg, Fiber: 6 g, Protein: 6 g, Carbohydrates: 12 g, Sodium: 565 mg*

GARLIC-STEAMED BROCCOLI RABE

Also known as broccoli raab or rapini, broccoli rabe is actually in the turnip family. Its flowers, leaves, and stalks are all edible and have a mildly bitter taste that is complemented here with lots of garlic and red pepper flakes.

- 2 tablespoons extra-virgin olive oil
- 1 tablespoon unsalted, grass-fed butter
- 3 garlic cloves, thinly sliced
- 2 bunches broccoli rabe, trimmed and cut into thirds
- ½ teaspoon crushed red pepper flakes
- 1 teaspoon sea salt

In a 12-inch skillet, warm the olive oil and butter over medium-high heat until the butter foams. Add the garlic and cook, stirring occasionally, until lightly browned, about 2 minutes. Add the broccoli rabe, toss to coat with the fat, and pour in ½ cup filtered water. Cover and cook until the broccoli rabe is tender, about 5 minutes.

Sprinkle the red pepper flakes and salt over the broccoli rabe, toss to combine, and serve.

Nutritional analysis per serving: Calories: 180, Fat: 16 g, Saturated Fat: 4 g, Cholesterol: 8 mg, Fiber: 3 g, Protein: 4 g, Carbohydrates: 4 g, Sodium: 606 mg

CREAMED TURMERIC KALE WITH RED BELL PEPPERS

Serves: 4

Prep time:
15 minutes

Cook time:
10 minutes

This is comfort food with a nutritional upgrade. Turmeric, an inflammation-fighting spice, pairs nicely with rich coconut cream. This simple dish is a unique and tasty way to enjoy kale.

- 2 tablespoons extra-virgin olive oil
- 2 garlic cloves, thinly sliced
- 2 red bell peppers, seeded and finely diced
- 2 bunches lacinato kale, stemmed and roughly chopped
- ¼ cup full-fat coconut milk
- 1 teaspoon ground turmeric
- ½ teaspoon sea salt

In a 10-inch skillet, warm the olive oil over medium heat until shimmering. Stir in the garlic and cook until fragrant, about 30 seconds. Add the bell peppers and cook, stirring occasionally, until just beginning to soften, about 2 minutes. Add the kale, toss with tongs to combine, and pour in the coconut milk. Stir in the turmeric and salt, cover, and cook, stirring occasionally, until the kale is wilted, 2 to 3 minutes. Serve.

Nutritional analysis per serving: Calories: 157, Fat: 8 g, Saturated Fat: 1 g, Cholesterol: 0 mg, Fiber: 3 g, Protein: 3 g, Carbohydrates: 12 g, Sodium: 307 mg

BRAISED COLLARD GREENS

Serves: 4

Prep time:
10 minutes

Cook time:
45 minutes

Collard greens might be one of the healthiest foods on the planet. The benefits of consuming them are too many to mention here, but a notable one is lowered cholesterol. If you're not familiar with collard greens, this recipe is the best introduction, as these collards are buttery and delicious.

- 2 tablespoons Ghee (page 279)
- 1 large yellow onion, thinly sliced
- 3 garlic cloves, minced
- 2 bunches collard greens, tough stems removed, leaves sliced
- 2 cups chicken or vegetable stock
- 1 teaspoon sea salt
- ¼ teaspoon freshly ground black pepper

In a large pot, warm the ghee over medium heat until shimmering. Add the onion and cook, stirring occasionally, until slightly softened, about 2 minutes. Stir in the garlic and cook until fragrant, about 1 minute. Add the collard greens and cook, stirring to combine, for 1 minute. Pour in the stock and bring to a simmer. Cover and cook until the greens are tender, about 40 minutes.

Stir the salt and pepper into the greens and serve.

Nutritional analysis per serving: *Calories: 135, Fat: 9 g, Saturated Fat: 5 g, Cholesterol: 4 mg, Fiber: 1 g, Protein: 4 g, Carbohydrates: 10 g, Sodium: 737 mg*

CELERY ROOT HASH

Serves: 4

Prep time:
10 minutes

Cook time:
20 minutes

Rich in vitamins A, C, K, and E, as well as in other nutrients, this celery root hash is comfort food that's good for you. It's the perfect side dish to just about any main course.

- 1 to 2 tablespoons extra-virgin olive oil
- 1 tablespoon unsalted, grass-fed butter
- 2 large celery roots, peeled and finely diced
- 1 small yellow onion, finely diced
- 2 sprigs rosemary, leaves only, finely chopped
- 1 teaspoon sea salt
- ¼ teaspoon freshly ground black pepper

In a large skillet, warm 1 tablespoon of the olive oil and the butter over medium heat until the butter melts. Add the celery root, toss to coat with fat, and cook, stirring occasionally, until slightly softened, 7 to 8 minutes. Stir in the onion and continue to cook until the celery root is tender, about 10 minutes, adding an additional 1 tablespoon oil if needed to prevent sticking.

Stir in the rosemary, salt, and pepper and serve.

Nutritional analysis per serving: *Calories: 117, Fat: 10 g, Saturated Fat: 3 g, Cholesterol: 8 mg, Fiber: 3 g, Protein: 1 g, Carbohydrates: 5 g, Sodium: 442 mg*

Zucchini "Noodles" with Shiitake Mushrooms and Ume Vinegar

Serves: 4

Prep time:
10 minutes

Cook time:
10 minutes

Umeboshi, also known simply as ume, are Japanese plumlike fruits that are traditionally preserved in salt. They have a long history of use as a digestive aid. The liquid that the fruits release during the salting process is referred to as ume vinegar, though it actually is not vinegar. Here, ume vinegar (found in most grocery stores' Asian sections) adds pleasing salty and acidic flavors to subtly sweet zucchini and earthy shiitake mushrooms.

- 2 large zucchini, ends trimmed
- 2 tablespoons sesame oil
- 2 garlic cloves, crushed
- 2 cups shiitake mushrooms, stemmed and sliced into ¼-inch strips
- 1 tablespoon ume vinegar
- 1 tablespoon toasted sesame oil
- 1 teaspoon crushed red pepper flakes
- 1 sheet nori, quartered and cut into thin strips

Using a spiral vegetable slicer (aka spiralizer) fitted with the shredder blade, cut the zucchini into spaghetti-size spiral strands. Use kitchen shears to cut the spirals into shorter lengths.

In a 10-inch skillet, warm the sesame oil over medium-high heat until shimmering. Add the garlic and mushrooms and cook, stirring frequently, until the mushrooms are softened and lightly browned, 3 to 4 minutes. Add the zucchini noodles, vinegar, toasted sesame oil, and red pepper flakes and cook, tossing to combine, until the noodles are just warmed through, about 3 minutes.

Divide the noodle mixture among 4 plates. Sprinkle each portion with nori strips and serve.

Nutritional analysis per serving: *Calories: 161, Fat: 11 g, Saturated Fat: 2 g, Cholesterol: 0 mg, Fiber: 0 g, Protein: 3 g, Carbohydrates: 14 g, Sodium: 445 mg*

STIR-FRIED BROCCOLI AND CABBAGE WITH GINGER-AVOCADO SAUCE

Serves: 4

Prep time:
15 minutes

Cook time:
20 minutes

Here's a vibrant stir-fry that can be made with whatever vegetables are fresh and in season. The rich and creamy avocado sauce is an unusual touch that adds great flavor and healthy fats to this meal.

- 1 (2-inch) piece ginger, peeled
- 2 avocados, pitted, peeled, and cut into large chunks
- 2 tablespoons fresh lime juice
- ¼ teaspoon sea salt
- ¼ teaspoon freshly ground black pepper
- 2 tablespoons coconut oil
- ¼ head cabbage (any kind), cored and shredded
- 1 small red onion, thinly sliced
- 2 garlic cloves, minced
- 1 large broccoli crown, stems peeled and cut into ¼-inch-thick rounds, florets cut into bite-size pieces
- 6 cups baby arugula
- ¼ cup toasted sesame seeds (optional)

To make the sauce, in a food processor, pulse the ginger until minced. Add the avocados, lime juice, salt, and pepper and process until smooth. With the machine running, pour in cold filtered water 1 to 2 tablespoons at a time, adding up to ½ cup, until the sauce is thick and creamy. Transfer to a bowl, cover, and refrigerate until ready to use.

In a large skillet or 10-inch wok, warm the coconut oil over medium heat until melted. Add the cabbage and onion and cook, stirring occasionally, until wilted and softened, 3 to 4 minutes. Stir in the garlic and cook until fragrant, about 1 minute. Add the broccoli, stir to combine, and pour in ¼ cup filtered water. Cover and cook until the broccoli is tender, about 3 minutes.

Divide the arugula among 4 plates and top with the stir-fry. Spoon about ¼ cup of the sauce over each portion, sprinkle with 1 tablespoon of the sesame seeds, if using, and serve.

Nutritional analysis per serving: *Calories: 357, Fat: 31 g, Saturated Fat: 9 g, Cholesterol: 0 mg, Fiber: 9 g, Protein: 6 g, Carbohydrates: 20 g, Sodium: 293 mg*

GINGER-TAMARI BAKED TOFU AND MUSHROOMS

Serves: 4

Prep time:
15 minutes, plus
marinating time

Cook time:
30 minutes

Tofu's neutral taste and ability to absorb flavors means you can infuse it with just about any seasonings you desire. Here it's marinated, along with earthy shiitake mushrooms, in Japanese staple ingredients for a deeply savory, umami-rich vegetarian main dish.

- 1 pound non-GMO firm tofu, drained
- 1 pound shiitake mushrooms, stemmed
- 2 tablespoons toasted sesame oil
- 1 tablespoon low-sodium, wheat-free tamari
- 2 tablespoons apple cider vinegar
- 1 tablespoon mirin
- 2 garlic cloves, minced
- 1 (1-inch) piece ginger, peeled and minced
- 1 teaspoon crushed red pepper flakes
- 2 scallions, thinly sliced

Place the tofu on a plate. Set another plate on top of the tofu and weigh it down with a large can (a 28-ounce can of tomatoes works nicely). Let stand at room temperature for 30 minutes.

Transfer the tofu to a cutting board and cut it into 8 evenly sized cubes. Combine the tofu cubes and the shiitake mushrooms in a glass baking dish.

In a bowl, stir together the sesame oil, tamari, vinegar, mirin, garlic, ginger, and red pepper flakes. Pour this mixture over the tofu and mushrooms and toss to coat. Cover and refrigerate for at least 1 hour or up to overnight.

Preheat the oven to 350°F. Line a baking sheet with parchment paper.

Remove the tofu and mushrooms from the marinade, placing them in a single layer on the prepared baking sheet. Bake for 15 minutes, then flip the tofu and mushrooms and continue to bake until the tofu is lightly browned and the mushrooms are slightly crisp at the edges, about 15 more minutes.

Transfer the tofu and mushrooms to a platter. Top with the scallions and serve.

Nutritional analysis per serving: *Calories: 247, Fat: 15 g, Saturated Fat: 4 g, Cholesterol: 0 mg, Fiber: 3 g, Protein: 18 g, Carbohydrates: 14 g, Sodium: 213 mg*

BAKED MARINATED TEMPEH WITH SHIITAKE-TURNIP-CHARD HASH

Serves: 4

Prep time:
20 minutes,
plus marinating
time

Cook time:
20 minutes

If you've never tried tempeh, this dish is a great introduction. Marinating and roasting the tempeh squares infuses them with bold, savory flavor that's complemented by the earthy vegetable hash.

- 2 (8-ounce) blocks organic, GMO-free tempeh, cut into a total of 8 squares
- ½ cup extra-virgin olive oil
- ¼ cup coconut aminos or wheat-free tamari
- 2 tablespoons balsamic vinegar
- 2 tablespoons apple cider vinegar
- 2 tablespoons whole-grain mustard
- 4 garlic cloves, minced
- ¼ teaspoon chipotle powder
- 2 tablespoons coconut oil
- 1 large turnip, peeled and finely diced
- 1 small red onion, minced
- 10 large shiitake mushrooms, stemmed and sliced into thirds
- 4 large Swiss chard leaves, stemmed and cut into bite-size pieces

Place the tempeh in a glass baking dish. In a bowl, whisk together the olive oil, coconut aminos, balsamic vinegar, cider vinegar, mustard, half of the minced garlic, and the chipotle powder. Pour this mixture over the tempeh, cover, and gently shake the baking dish to coat the tempeh. Refrigerate for at least 8 hours or up to overnight, turning the tempeh pieces once or twice.

Preheat the oven to 350°F.

Remove the tempeh from the refrigerator and uncover. Place the baking dish in the oven and bake until the tempeh pieces are browned on the bottom, about 15 minutes.

Meanwhile, in a 10-inch skillet, warm 1 tablespoon of the coconut oil over medium heat until melted. Add the turnip and onion and cook, stirring occasionally, until the turnip begins to soften, about 5 minutes. Add the mushrooms, remaining coconut oil, and remaining garlic and cook, stirring occasionally, until the turnip is tender, 8 to 10 minutes. Stir in the Swiss chard and cook until the leaves are wilted.

Divide the vegetable hash among 4 plates, then top each portion with 2 pieces of tempeh. Drizzle the marinade remaining in the baking dish over the top and serve.

Nutritional analysis per serving: *Calories: 563, Fat: 42 g, Saturated Fat: 11 g, Cholesterol: 0 mg, Fiber: 12 g, Protein: 25 g, Carbohydrates: 29 g, Sodium: 1065 mg*

Tempeh and Bell Peppers with Tomato and Cardamom

Serves: 4

Prep time:
10 minutes

Cook time:
20 minutes

Cardamom is a warm, fragrant spice from a plant native to India, and it's commonly used in that country's cuisine. This dish, paired with Cauliflower "Rice" with Scallions (page 156), makes a great vegetarian meal.

- 1 tablespoon Ghee (page 279)
- 1 (8-ounce) block organic, non-GMO tempeh, cut into ½-inch chunks
- 1 large red onion, finely diced
- 1 red bell pepper, seeded and finely diced
- 1 green bell pepper, seeded and finely diced
- 2 teaspoons ground cardamom
- 2 garlic cloves, minced
- 1 cup tomato puree
- 1 cup vegetable stock or filtered water
- ½ teaspoon sea salt
- ½ cup loosely packed fresh cilantro leaves, roughly chopped

In a large skillet, warm the ghee over medium heat until melted. Add the tempeh and onion, toss to combine, and cook until the onion begins to soften, 2 to 3 minutes. Add the bell peppers and cook, stirring occasionally, until the peppers begin to soften, 2 to 3 minutes. Stir in the cardamom and garlic and cook until fragrant, about 1 minute. Pour in the tomato puree and stock and stir to combine. Cover and simmer, stirring occasionally, until all the liquid has been absorbed, 15 to 20 minutes.

Stir in the salt and cilantro and serve.

Nutritional analysis per serving: *Calories: 186, Fat: 7 g, Saturated Fat: 3 g, Cholesterol: 0 mg, Fiber: 8 g, Protein: 13 g, Carbohydrates: 19 g, Sodium: 333 mg*

TEMPEH, VEGETABLE, AND KELP NOODLE STIR-FRY

Serves: 4

Prep time:
20 minutes

Cook time:
10 minutes

If you've never tried kelp noodles, they will become a family favorite. A great alternative to wheat and rice noodles, they're the perfect addition to any stir-fry.

- 3 tablespoons sesame oil
- 1 (8-ounce) block organic, non-GMO tempeh, cut into eighths
- 1 small yellow onion, thinly sliced
- 1 large carrot, scrubbed and thinly sliced on the bias
- 2 cups (1-inch) broccoli florets
- 2 cups thinly sliced napa cabbage
- 1 (1-inch) piece ginger, peeled and minced
- ½ cup chicken or vegetable stock
- 3 tablespoons wheat-free tamari
- 1 pound kelp noodles, cut into 4-inch lengths and rinsed
- 1 bunch scallions, green parts only, thinly sliced

In a 10-inch skillet, warm 1 tablespoon of the sesame oil over medium-high heat until shimmering. Add the tempeh and cook until browned, about 2 minutes, then flip and cook for an additional 1 to 2 minutes. Transfer to a plate. Add the remaining 2 tablespoons sesame oil to the skillet and heat until shimmering. Add the onion, carrot, broccoli, and cabbage and cook, stirring occasionally, until the vegetables are slightly softened, 3 to 4 minutes. Stir in the ginger, stock, tamari, and tempeh, then remove the pan from the heat.

While the tempeh and vegetables cook, in a medium saucepan, bring 4 cups filtered water to a simmer over medium-high heat. Add the kelp noodles and cook just until heated through, about 3 minutes. Drain the noodles in a colander.

Add the noodles to the skillet, return the skillet to medium-high heat, and toss until the noodles are well combined with the tempeh and vegetables. Toss in the scallion greens and serve.

Nutritional analysis per serving: *Calories: 265, Fat: 14 g, Saturated Fat: 2 g, Cholesterol: 1 mg, Fiber: 7 g, Protein: 15 g, Carbohydrates: 20 g, Sodium: 680 mg*

11

Seafood

TAMARI AND ORANGE-MARINATED COD WITH BOK CHOY

Serves: 4

Prep time: 10 minutes, plus marinating time

Cook time: 15 minutes

PEGAN DIET

Here's a simple but wholesome fish-and-vegetable dish that requires minimal prep and cooks in only 15 minutes, making it a perfect weeknight meal. The bold character of citrus and tamari complements the clean flavor of the cod.

- 2 tablespoons low-sodium, wheat-free tamari
- 1 tablespoon fish sauce
- 1 tablespoon rice vinegar
- ¼ cup fresh orange juice
- 1 (1-inch) piece ginger, peeled and minced
- 4 (4-ounce) cod fillets
- 1 tablespoon sesame oil
- 2 garlic cloves, minced
- 1 large head bok choy, cut crosswise into 1-inch pieces, rinsed and drained

In an 8-inch square glass baking dish, stir together 1 tablespoon of the tamari and the fish sauce, vinegar, orange juice, and ginger. Add the cod fillets in a single layer and flip them over several times to coat with the marinade. Cover and refrigerate for 30 minutes.

Preheat the oven to 350°F.

Transfer the fish to a clean baking dish, placing the fillets in a single layer, and bake until the flesh is firm and flakes easily, about 8 minutes.

While the fish cooks, in a 10-inch skillet, warm the sesame oil over medium-high heat until shimmering. Add the garlic and cook, stirring frequently, until lightly browned, about 1 minute. Stir in the bok choy, then pour in ¼ cup filtered water and the remaining tamari. Cover and cook until the bok choy stems are tender-crisp, 2 to 3 minutes.

Divide the bok choy among 4 plates, top each portion with a cod fillet, and serve.

Nutritional analysis per serving: *Calories: 182, Fat: 5 g, Saturated Fat: 1 g, Cholesterol: 0 mg, Fiber: 0 g, Protein: 27 g, Carbohydrates: 5 g, Sodium: 791 mg*

BAKED HADDOCK WITH FENNEL-CAULIFLOWER PUREE

Serves: 4

Prep time:
20 minutes

Cook time:
20 minutes

This is a simple but elegant dish. The fennel imparts a sweet and earthy flavor to the cauliflower and adds an herbal aroma to the fish as it bakes.

- 1 head cauliflower, trimmed
- 2 tablespoons extra-virgin olive oil
- 3 tablespoons unsalted, grass-fed butter
- 1 large leek, white section halved lengthwise, rinsed well, and thinly sliced
- 1 large fennel bulb, fronds reserved, bulb cut in half, cored, and roughly chopped
- 2 garlic cloves, minced
- 1 cup chicken stock
- 2 (8-ounce) skinless haddock fillets
- 1 teaspoon sea salt
- ½ teaspoon freshly ground black pepper

Preheat the oven to 350°F.

Using a chef's knife, cut the head of cauliflower in half, then use a paring knife to cut the florets away from the core; discard the core. Cut the florets into rough 1-inch pieces.

In a large Dutch oven or stockpot, warm 1 tablespoon of the olive oil and 1 tablespoon of the butter over medium heat until the butter melts. Add the leek and fennel and cook, stirring occasionally, until softened but not at all browned, about 5 minutes. Stir in the garlic and cook until fragrant, about 2–3 minutes. Add the cauliflower and stir to combine. Pour in the chicken stock, cover, and simmer, stirring occasionally, until the vegetables are completely tender, about 10 minutes.

Meanwhile, lay half of the fennel fronds on a rimmed baking sheet. Place the fish on top of the fronds, drizzle the fillets with the remaining 1 tablespoon olive oil, and sprinkle with ½ teaspoon of the salt and ¼ teaspoon of the pepper. Top the fillets with the remaining fennel fronds. Bake the fish until just firm to the touch and opaque throughout, 10 to

12 minutes. Remove from the oven and carefully scrape away the fennel fronds on top. Cut each fillet in half crosswise.

When the vegetables are tender, transfer the contents of the pot to a food processor. Add the remaining butter, the remaining salt, and the remaining pepper. Puree until smooth, scraping down the bowl as needed, about 1 minute. Return the puree to the pot and cover to keep warm.

Divide the vegetable puree among 4 plates and top each portion with a piece of fish. Serve.

Nutritional analysis per serving: *Calories: 346, Fat: 18 g, Saturated Fat: 7 g, Cholesterol: 119 mg, Fiber: 4 g, Protein: 33 g, Carbohydrates: 13 g, Sodium: 860 mg*

LEMON-BAKED SOLE WITH STEWED SUMMER SQUASH

Serves: 4

Prep time:
20 minutes

Cook time:
25 minutes

Sole is a delicate whitefish that pairs well with a wide range of ingredients. Here, I combine sole with fresh summer squash, herbs, and arugula for a light, healthful meal.

- 3 tablespoons extra-virgin olive oil
- 4 (6-ounce) skinless sole or flounder fillets
- 2 teaspoons chopped fresh thyme
- ½ teaspoon sea salt
- ½ teaspoon freshly ground black pepper
- ½ small red onion, very thinly sliced
- 1 lemon, sliced into thin circles
- 1 tablespoon Ghee (page 279)
- 2 yellow summer squash, cut into ¼-inch-thick rounds
- 3 garlic cloves, minced
- 2 teaspoons dried oregano
- 1 large tomato, roughly chopped
- 4 cups baby arugula

Preheat the oven to 350°F.

Drizzle 1 tablespoon of the olive oil into a baking dish large enough to hold the fish in a single layer. Lay the fillets in the baking dish and sprinkle them evenly with the thyme, a pinch of salt, and ¼ teaspoon of the pepper. Scatter the onion slices over the top, then drizzle with 1 tablespoon of the remaining olive oil. Lay the lemon slices on top of the fillets. Set aside.

In a 12-inch skillet, warm the remaining olive oil and the ghee over medium-high heat until shimmering. Add the squash slices, toss gently, and cook, stirring occasionally, until the squash begins to soften, about 3 minutes. Stir in the garlic, oregano, and remaining salt.

Place the fish in the oven and bake until the fillets are just firm to the touch and opaque throughout, 6 to 8 minutes. While the fish bakes, continue to cook the squash, stirring occasionally, until tender.

After removing the fish from the oven, add the tomato to the skillet with the squash, toss to combine, and cook until the tomato is just warmed through, 1 to 2 minutes.

Divide the arugula among 4 plates and spoon the summer squash mixture on top. Carefully place a fish fillet with the onions and lemon slices on each portion of squash and serve.

Nutritional analysis per serving: *Calories: 445, Fat: 33 g, Saturated Fat: 7 g, Cholesterol: 93 mg, Fiber: 3 g, Protein: 31 g, Carbohydrates: 7 g, Sodium: 320 mg*

Coconut Sole with Black Beans and Spinach

Serves: 4

Prep time:
5 minutes

Cook time:
15 minutes

PEGAN DIET

Everyone should have a few healthful one-pot meals like this one in his or her repertoire for those days when dinner needs to be on the table in an instant. This delicious Mexican-influenced dish is loaded with flavor but can be prepared in only 20 minutes.

- 2 tablespoons coconut oil
- 1 large yellow onion, thinly sliced
- 1 (15-ounce) can black beans, rinsed and drained
- 1 teaspoon ground cumin
- 1 teaspoon ground coriander
- ¾ teaspoon sea salt
- ¼ cup full-fat coconut milk
- 12 cups baby spinach
- 4 (4-ounce) skinless sole or flounder fillets
- juice of ½ lime

In a 10-inch skillet, warm the coconut oil over medium heat until melted. Add the onion and cook, stirring occasionally, until softened, 2 to 3 minutes. Add the beans, cumin, coriander, and a pinch of the salt and stir to combine. Pour in the coconut milk and bring to a simmer. Scatter the spinach in an even layer in the pan and use your hands to slightly flatten the leaves. Lay the fish in a single layer on top of the spinach, sprinkle the fillets with the remaining salt, and squeeze the juice from the lime half over the top. Cover and cook until the fish is opaque throughout, 4 to 5 minutes.

Divide the fish, spinach, and bean mixture among 4 plates and serve.

Nutritional analysis per serving: *Calories: 309, Fat: 11 g, Saturated Fat: 9 g, Cholesterol: 62 mg, Fiber: 7 g, Protein: 27 g, Carbohydrates: 24 g, Sodium: 855 mg*

SAUTÉED PERCH WITH TOMATO-MANGO SALSA

PEGAN DIET

Perch is a freshwater fish with a delicate texture similar to that of sole or flounder. The small size of the fillets means they cook up in a matter of just a few minutes. Here, a colorful, tangy-sweet salsa is the perfect pairing for perch's mild flavor.

Serves: 4

Prep time: 20 minutes

Cook time: 15 minutes

- 1 mango, peeled and cut into ¼-inch dice
- 1 large tomato, cut into ¼-inch dice
- ½ cup fresh cilantro leaves, roughly chopped
- grated zest and juice of 1 lime
- ¼ cup extra-virgin olive oil
- 1 small jalapeño, seeded and minced
- 8 (2-ounce) skin-on perch fillets
- 1 teaspoon sea salt
- 1 teaspoon ground cumin
- ¼ teaspoon freshly ground black pepper
- 2 tablespoons Ghee (page 279)

In a bowl, combine the mango, tomato, cilantro, lime zest and juice, olive oil, and jalapeño. Mix well, then let stand to allow the flavors to mingle while you prepare the fish.

Season the perch fillets with the salt, cumin, and pepper. In a large skillet, warm the ghee over medium-high heat until shimmering. Lay the fillets flesh side down in a single layer in the skillet and cook until halfway done, about 3 minutes. Using a metal spatula, flip the fillets, turn off the heat, and allow the fish to finish cooking with the pan's residual heat, about 2 minutes.

Transfer 2 fillets to each of 4 plates. Top each portion with the salsa and serve.

Nutritional analysis per serving: *Calories: 538, Fat: 29 g, Saturated Fat: 8 g, Cholesterol: 111 mg, Fiber: 6 g, Protein: 47 g, Carbohydrates: 25 g, Sodium: 1377 mg*

BAKED HALIBUT WITH BUTTERNUT SQUASH–CARROT PUREE

Serves: 4

Prep time:
10 minutes

Cook time:
20 minutes

In addition to being amazingly delicious, this simple dish is incredibly good for you. Butternut squash is rich in fiber, antioxidants, and phytonutrients; carrots are loaded with beta-carotene; and halibut is rich in omega-3 fats.

- 2 tablespoons coconut oil
- 1 scallion, thinly sliced
- 2 carrots, scrubbed and cut into 1-inch pieces
- 1 small butternut squash, peeled, seeded, and cut into 1-inch cubes
- 3 tablespoons coconut butter
- 2 tablespoons apple cider vinegar
- 2 teaspoons sea salt
- 2 teaspoons chopped fresh thyme
- 2 teaspoons paprika
- ¼ teaspoon freshly ground black pepper
- 1½ pounds halibut fillets (or other lean whitefish such as haddock or cod)
- 2 tablespoons extra-virgin olive oil

Preheat the oven to 350°F.

In a large saucepan, warm the coconut oil over medium heat until melted. Add the scallion and cook, stirring occasionally, until softened, about 2 minutes. Add the carrots and butternut squash, stir to combine, then pour in ½ cup filtered water. Cover and cook until the vegetables are completely tender, 6 to 7 minutes.

Transfer the vegetables to a food processor and pulse a few times to break down the pieces. Add the coconut butter, vinegar, and 1 teaspoon of the salt and process until the mixture has the consistency of mashed potatoes, about 30 seconds. Return the puree to the saucepan and cover to keep warm.

In a small bowl, stir together the thyme, paprika, pepper, and remaining salt. Coat the fish fillets all over with the olive oil, then rub with the thyme mixture. Place the fish in a single layer in a baking dish and bake until opaque throughout, 8 to 10 minutes.

Divide the vegetable puree among 4 plates, top each portion with a piece of fish, and serve.

Nutritional analysis per serving: Calories: 432, Fat: 32 g, Saturated Fat: 20 g, Cholesterol: 0 mg, Fiber: 4 g, Protein: 28 g, Carbohydrates: 11 g, Sodium: 677 mg

ARCTIC CHAR WITH SWISS CHARD AND MUSTARD VINAIGRETTE

Serves: 4

Prep time: 15 minutes

Cook time: 15 minutes

According to seafood watch lists, Arctic char is sustainable and therefore a good choice for eco-conscious consumers. The pink-fleshed cold-water fish can be prepared in the same ways as salmon, its close relative. Swiss chard contains numerous polyphenols that have been shown to help regulate blood sugar, and that's just one of the vegetable's many benefits.

- ¼ cup plus 2 tablespoons extra-virgin olive oil
- 2 tablespoons apple cider vinegar
- 1½ tablespoons whole-grain mustard
- 4 (4-ounce) skin-on Arctic char fillets
- 1 teaspoon, plus pinch sea salt
- ½ teaspoon freshly ground black pepper
- 1 tablespoon Ghee (page 279)
- 2 bunches Swiss chard, stemmed, leaves cut into bite-size pieces
- slice of lemon and sprinkle of fresh parsley, for garnish (optional)

To make the mustard vinaigrette, in a small bowl, whisk together ¼ cup of the olive oil and the vinegar and mustard. Set the vinaigrette aside.

Season the fish with 1 teaspoon of salt and the pepper. In a large cast-iron skillet, warm the ghee over medium-high heat until shimmering. Carefully place the fish flesh side down in the pan and cook until halfway done, about 4 minutes. Using a metal spatula, flip each piece, turn off the heat, and allow the fish to finish cooking with the pan's residual heat, about 2 minutes.

While the fish cooks, in a second large skillet, warm the remaining olive oil over medium-high heat until shimmering. Add the Swiss chard and a pinch of salt. Using tongs, toss the chard and cook until completely wilted, about 3 minutes.

Divide the chard among 4 plates and top each portion with a fish fillet. Whisk the vinaigrette to recombine, drizzle the chard and fish with the vinaigrette, and serve garnished with the lemon and parsley, if using.

Nutritional analysis per serving: *Calories: 405, Fat: 30 g, Saturated Fat: 9 g, Cholesterol: 32 mg, Fiber: 1 g, Protein: 25 g, Carbohydrates: 1 g, Sodium: 854 mg*

DILL BUTTER-BAKED SALMON WITH BEET AND ROASTED PEPPER SALAD

Serves: 4

Prep time:
10 minutes

Cook time:
20 minutes

When it comes to fish, wild salmon is my top choice. Because salmon contains large amounts of omega-3 fatty acids, it is widely regarded as a superfood. A 4-ounce piece of baked or broiled salmon contains at least 2 grams of omega-3 fats! So if you're looking to add more omega-3s to your diet, try this buttery baked salmon with a delicious beet salad accompaniment. I prefer the flavor and texture of salmon when the center of the fillet is still slightly translucent, but you can cook the fillets until done to your liking.

- 3 large beets, peeled and finely diced
- 2 large jarred roasted red peppers, sliced into thin strips
- 1 shallot, sliced into thin rounds
- ¼ cup loosely packed fresh parsley leaves, roughly chopped
- 1½ tablespoons balsamic vinegar
- 3 tablespoons extra-virgin olive oil
- ½ teaspoon sea salt
- ½ teaspoon freshly ground black pepper
- 4 (4-ounce) wild salmon fillets
- 8 tablespoons unsalted, grass-fed butter, at room temperature
- ¼ cup fresh dill leaves, roughly chopped
- 1 lemon, halved and seeded

Preheat the oven to 350°F.

Place the beets in a saucepan and cover with filtered water. Bring to a boil over high heat, then reduce the heat to maintain a simmer and cook until the beets are tender, about 10 minutes. Drain the beets, submerge them in a bowl of cold water until cooled, and drain again.

In a bowl, combine the beets, roasted peppers, shallot, parsley, balsamic vinegar, olive oil, sea salt, and ¼ teaspoon of the pepper. Mix well, then set aside.

Coat a baking dish large enough to hold the salmon in a single layer with 1 tablespoon of the butter, then place the fillets in the dish. In a small bowl, combine the remaining butter, the dill, and the remaining ¼ teaspoon pepper and mix with a spoon until well combined. Spread the dill butter on the salmon fillets, dividing it evenly. Squeeze the juice from the lemon halves over the salmon. Bake the salmon until the fish is firm but the very center of the fillets is still translucent, 8 to 10 minutes.

Divide the salad among 4 plates. Place a salmon fillet on each plate and serve.

Nutritional analysis per serving: *Calories: 520, Fat: 43 g, Saturated Fat: 21 g, Cholesterol: 174 mg, Fiber: 3 g, Protein: 25 g, Carbohydrates: 10 g, Sodium: 776 mg*

SALMON WITH RED CABBAGE AND ORANGE SALAD

Serves: 4

Prep time:
15 minutes

Cook time:
10 minutes

PEGAN DIET

A sweet-and-sour salad offsets the fattiness of wild salmon, my favorite fish. This dish is so fresh and filled with vibrant colors, making it pleasing for the eyes and stomach. I prefer the flavor and texture of salmon when it's a little underdone—that is, when the center of the fillet is still slightly translucent—but cook the fillets until done to your liking.

- 4 (4- to 5-ounce) skin-on wild salmon fillets
- 4 tablespoons extra-virgin olive oil
- 1 teaspoon sea salt
- ¼ teaspoon freshly ground black pepper
- 2 oranges
- 1 small head red cabbage, cored and shredded
- ¼ cup loosely packed mint leaves, chopped
- ¼ cup loosely packed basil leaves, chopped
- 2 tablespoons rice vinegar

Preheat the oven to 350°F.

Place the salmon in a baking dish large enough to hold the fillets in a single layer. Drizzle with 2 tablespoons of the olive oil and sprinkle with ½ teaspoon of the salt and the pepper. Rub the oil and seasonings all over the fillets. Bake until the salmon is firm to the touch, 8 to 10 minutes.

While the fish bakes, cut off the top and bottom of an orange. Stand the orange on a cut side and, using a sharp knife, cut away the rind and white pith in strips from top to bottom, following the contour of the fruit. Lay the orange on its side and cut it into ¼-inch-thick rounds. Repeat with the remaining orange.

In a large bowl, combine the orange rounds, cabbage, mint, basil, vinegar, remaining 2 tablespoons oil, and remaining salt. Toss until well mixed.

Place a salmon fillet on each of 4 plates. Divide the salad among the plates and serve.

Nutritional analysis per serving: *Calories: 410, Fat: 25 g, Saturated Fat: 8 g, Cholesterol: 128 mg, Fiber: 5 g, Protein: 28 g, Carbohydrates: 21 g, Sodium: 704 mg*

KIMCHI AND SWEET POTATO FISH CAKES WITH CABBAGE-APPLE SLAW

Serves: 4

Prep time:
30 minutes

Cook time:
10 minutes

PEGAN DIET

Here, spicy, garlicky kimchi is tempered by mashed sweet potatoes and mild-flavored whitefish. You can prep the fish cakes the night before and then cook them and make the slaw when you're ready to serve dinner.

- 1 small head red cabbage, shredded
- 1 Granny Smith apple, cored and julienned
- 1 red bell pepper, seeded and julienned
- ½ cup loosely packed fresh cilantro leaves, roughly chopped
- 2 tablespoons fresh mint leaves, roughly chopped
- 2 tablespoons rice vinegar
- 2 tablespoons extra-virgin olive oil
- 1 teaspoon sea salt
- 1½ pounds haddock fillets
- 8 ounces sweet potatoes, peeled and cut into 1-inch chunks
- 2 tablespoons unsalted, grass-fed butter
- ½ cup drained kimchi, roughly chopped
- 2 scallions, thinly sliced
- 1 large egg, beaten
- 3 tablespoons coconut flour
- coconut oil, for cooking
- 1 lime, cut into 8 wedges

In a large bowl, combine the cabbage, apple, and bell pepper and toss to combine. Add the cilantro, mint, vinegar, 1 tablespoon of the olive oil, and ½ teaspoon of the salt. Mix until thoroughly combined. Cover and refrigerate until you're ready to serve.

In a large skillet, warm the remaining olive oil over medium-high heat until shimmering. Carefully add the fish and cook for 3 minutes, then flip the fillets. Cover, reduce the heat to medium, and continue to cook until the fillets are opaque and firm, 3 to 4 more minutes. Transfer the fish to a plate and allow to cool.

Place the sweet potatoes in a small saucepan and pour in 1 cup filtered water. Cover, bring to a simmer over medium-high heat, and cook until the sweet potatoes are completely tender, about 8 minutes. Drain the sweet potatoes in a colander and return them to the saucepan. Add the butter and, using a potato masher, smash the sweet potatoes, keeping them slightly chunky.

Transfer the sweet potatoes to a bowl and gently fold in the fish, kimchi, scallions, egg, and coconut flour. Stir in the remaining salt. Form the mixture into 8 evenly sized patties, each about 2 inches in diameter and 1 inch thick.

In a large skillet, warm 2 tablespoons coconut oil over medium-high heat until shimmering. Carefully add the fish cakes and cook until lightly browned, about 3 minutes. Flip the fish cakes, add more coconut oil if the pan is dry, and continue to cook until the second sides are lightly browned and the cakes are heated through, about 3 more minutes.

Arrange 2 fish cakes on each of 4 plates and mound the slaw alongside. Place 2 lime wedges on each plate and serve.

Nutritional analysis per serving: *Calories: 622, Fat: 31 g, Saturated Fat: 16 g, Cholesterol: 204 mg, Fiber: 9 g, Protein: 47 g, Carbohydrates: 28 g, Sodium: 917 mg*

Shrimp Scampi

Serves: 4

Prep time:
15 minutes

Cook time:
15 minutes

This version of the Italian American classic will become a favorite in your household. Shrimp have a high EPA and DHA content, so they're great for heart health and nervous system support. Serve this dish solo or with gluten-free spaghetti when you're off the twenty-one-day plan.

- 4 tablespoons extra-virgin olive oil
- 1 pound large shrimp, peeled and deveined
- 1 large yellow onion, thinly sliced
- 1 tablespoon minced garlic
- 1 large tomato, roughly chopped
- ½ cup white wine
- 1 teaspoon sea salt
- ¼ teaspoon freshly ground black pepper
- 2 tablespoons unsalted, grass-fed butter
- ¼ cup fresh parsley leaves, roughly chopped

In a large skillet, heat 2 tablespoons of the olive oil over medium-high heat until shimmering. Add the shrimp in an even layer and cook without stirring until lightly browned, about 1 minute. Flip each shrimp and continue to cook until lightly browned on the second sides, about 1 more minute; the shrimp may not be fully cooked at this point, but that's okay. Transfer the shrimp to a plate and set aside.

Return the pan to medium-high heat and add the remaining 2 tablespoons olive oil. Add the onion and garlic and cook, stirring occasionally, until the onion begins to soften, about 3 minutes. Add the tomato, stir to combine, then pour in the wine and simmer until slightly reduced. Add ¼ cup filtered water and continue to simmer until the sauce is reduced by half, about 8 minutes.

Add the shrimp to the sauce, toss gently to coat, and cook until the shrimp are opaque throughout, 2 to 3 minutes. Season with the salt and pepper, stir in the butter and parsley, and serve.

Nutritional analysis per serving: *Calories: 326, Fat: 21 g, Saturated Fat: 6 g, Cholesterol: 236 mg, Fiber: 1 g, Protein: 25 g, Carbohydrates: 6 g, Sodium: 851 mg*

SHRIMP WITH SWEET POTATOES, KALE, AND COCONUT MILK

Serves: 4

Prep time:
15 minutes

Cook time:
10 minutes

This is a super-simple yet deeply nourishing one-pot recipe that combines good-quality fats from coconut milk, ghee, and shrimp with nutrient-dense veggies and healing spices.

- 2 tablespoons Ghee (page 279)
- 2 large sweet potatoes, peeled and finely diced
- 2 tablespoons peeled and grated ginger
- 2 teaspoons ground turmeric
- 1 cup full-fat coconut milk
- 1 pound large shrimp, peeled and deveined
- 1 small bunch lacinato kale, stemmed and roughly chopped
- 1 teaspoon sea salt
- 2 tablespoons fresh lime juice
- ½ cup fresh cilantro leaves

In a 10-inch skillet, warm the ghee over medium-high heat until shimmering. Add the sweet potatoes, toss to coat with fat, and cook until almost tender, 3 to 4 minutes. Stir in the ginger and turmeric, then pour in the coconut milk. Bring to a simmer, then add the shrimp and scatter the kale on top. Cover and cook until the shrimp are opaque throughout and the kale is wilted, about 3 minutes. Stir in the salt and lime juice.

Divide the shrimp, vegetables, and sauce evenly into 4 bowls. Garnish with the cilantro and serve.

Nutritional analysis per serving: *Calories: 486, Fat: 30 g, Saturated Fat: 23 g, Cholesterol: 221 mg, Fiber: 5 g, Protein: 29 g, Carbohydrates: 27 g, Sodium: 929 mg*

SCALLOPS MEUNIÈRE

Serves: 4

Prep time:
15 minutes

Cook time:
10 minutes

In classic French cooking, meunière is a preparation of sautéed flour–dredged fish with browned butter, lemon, and parsley. This spin puts coconut flour on scallops and includes lemon slices in the buttery sauce. This is a great dish to serve on date night.

- ½ cup coconut flour
- 1 teaspoon sea salt
- ½ teaspoon freshly ground black pepper
- 12 large sea scallops (about 1 pound), side muscles removed, patted dry
- 8 tablespoons unsalted, grass-fed butter
- 1 lemon, cut into ¼-inch slices
- ½ cup fresh parsley leaves, roughly chopped

In a bowl, whisk together the coconut flour, salt, and pepper. Working two or three at a time, dredge the scallops in the seasoned flour, shake off the excess, and place on a plate.

In a large skillet, warm 2 tablespoons of the butter over medium-high heat until foaming. Add half of the scallops and cook until golden brown, about 3 minutes. Flip each scallop and cook just until firm, about 1 more minute; do not overcook or the scallops will become rubbery. Transfer the scallops to a platter and cover with aluminum foil to keep warm. Add 2 tablespoons of the remaining butter to the skillet and cook the remaining scallops in the same way.

Wipe out the skillet, set it over medium-high heat, and add the remaining butter. Add the lemon slices and cook until they begin to soften, about 2 minutes. Stir in the parsley.

Pour the sauce (including the lemon slices) over the scallops and serve.

Nutritional analysis per serving: *Calories: 166, Fat: 3 g, Saturated Fat: 2 g, Cholesterol: 35 mg, Fiber: 5 g, Protein: 21 g, Carbohydrates: 12 g, Sodium: 854 mg*

SEARED SCALLOPS WITH CURRIED BRUSSELS SPROUT SLAW

Serves: 4

Prep time: 30 minutes

Cook time: 5 minutes

Scallops have a sweet, buttery flavor that I love, and as an added bonus, they are an excellent source of protein and fat. This dish is elevated comfort food that's both easy to prepare and amazingly delicious.

- 1 cup Homemade Mayonnaise (page 265)
- 1 tablespoon curry powder
- 1 tablespoon apple cider vinegar
- ½ teaspoon freshly ground black pepper
- 1 pound Brussels sprouts, trimmed
- 1 large carrot, scrubbed and grated
- 4 scallions, green parts only, thinly sliced
- ½ cup toasted walnuts, roughly chopped
- 1 teaspoon sea salt
- 12 large sea scallops (about 1 pound), side muscles removed, patted dry
- 2 tablespoons Ghee (page 279)
- 1 lemon, cut into four wedges

In a small bowl, whisk together the mayonnaise, curry powder, vinegar, and ¼ teaspoon of the pepper. Set aside.

Using a mandolin, a food processor fitted with a slicing disk, or a sharp knife, slice the Brussels sprouts as thinly as possible, then place in a large bowl. Add the carrot, scallions, walnuts, and mayonnaise mixture and stir until well combined. Season with ½ teaspoon of the salt, then set aside.

Season the scallops with the remaining salt and the remaining pepper. In a large skillet, warm the ghee over high heat until shimmering. Add the scallops to the pan in a single layer and cook until golden brown, about 3 minutes. Using tongs, carefully flip each scallop and cook for 1 more minute; do not overcook or the scallops will become rubbery.

Place 3 scallops on each of 4 plates and spoon the slaw alongside. Serve with the lemon wedges.

Nutritional analysis per serving: *Calories: 456, Fat: 19 g, Saturated Fat: 5 g, Cholesterol: 0 mg, Fiber: 7 g, Protein: 34 g, Carbohydrates: 17 g, Sodium: 808 mg*

COCONUT-SIMMERED SCALLOPS WITH QUICK-PICKLED VEGETABLES

Serves: 4

Prep time:
30 minutes

Cook time:
10 minutes

Creamy, with a little bit of heat and the perfect amount of tartness from fresh lime juice, this quick-cooking dish packs a lot of flavor. The crisp, tangy, "pickled" vegetables contrast pleasantly with the tender scallops and rich sauce. Because the scallops are in thin slices and begin to "cook" in the acidic marinade, take extra care not to overcook them on the stove top.

- 1 pound large sea scallops, side muscles removed, cut in half across the grain
- ½ cup full-fat coconut milk
- 2 tablespoons fresh lime juice
- 4 teaspoons fish sauce
- 2 teaspoons ground coriander
- 1 small jalapeño, sliced into thin rounds
- 2 cups of snap peas, cut into thirds on the bias
- 1 large red bell pepper, seeded and cut into thin strips
- 1 large cucumber, trimmed and sliced into ¼-inch rounds
- 2 tablespoons rice vinegar
- 1 tablespoon toasted sesame oil
- 1 tablespoon extra-virgin olive oil
- ½ teaspoon sea salt
- ½ cup roughly chopped unsalted roasted cashews

Place the scallops in a glass baking dish and add the coconut milk, lime juice, fish sauce, coriander, and jalapeño. Gently stir with a fork, then set aside to marinate while you prepare the vegetables.

Place the snap peas, bell pepper strips, and cucumber rounds in a large bowl. Add the vinegar, sesame oil, olive oil, and salt and toss until well combined. Set aside for 20 to 30 minutes to pickle.

Heat a medium skillet over medium heat for 2 minutes, then pour in the scallops along with the marinade. Cook, stirring gently and occasionally, until the scallops are just opaque throughout, about 5 minutes; do not overcook.

Divide the scallops and sauce among 4 plates, then spoon the vegetables alongside. Sprinkle with the cashews and serve.

Nutritional analysis per serving: Calories: 363, Fat: 24 g, Saturated Fat: 7 g, Cholesterol: 37 mg, Fiber: 2 g, Protein: 23 g, Carbohydrates: 17 g, Sodium: 706 mg

THAI RED CURRY WITH SEAFOOD AND VEGETABLES

Serves: 4

Prep time:
20 minutes

Cook time:
25 minutes

I love Thai curry but I resist ordering it in restaurants because of the sugar it contains. So I was determined to include a recipe in this book for Thai curry that's suitable for the *Eat Fat, Get Thin* Plan. My version is filled with all the requisite big, bold flavors, as well as with phytonutrients from the broccoli, peppers, and cilantro. It will not disappoint!

- 2 tablespoons avocado oil
- 1 small onion, cut into large dice
- 1 large carrot, scrubbed and cut into ¼-inch rounds
- 1 (2-inch) piece ginger, peeled and grated
- 3 garlic cloves, minced
- 2 tablespoons Thai red curry paste
- 1 (13.5-ounce) can full-fat coconut milk
- 1 tablespoon fish sauce
- 1 large red bell pepper, seeded and sliced into ¼-inch strips
- 1 small broccoli crown, stems peeled and cut into thin rounds, florets cut into bite-size pieces
- 8 ounces large shrimp, peeled, deveined, and cut into thirds
- 8 ounces sea scallops, side muscles removed, cut horizontally into thin rounds
- 1 pound mussels, scrubbed and debearded
- ½ cup packed fresh cilantro leaves, roughly chopped
- 1 lime, cut into 4 wedges

In a 10-inch skillet, warm the avocado oil over medium–high heat until shimmering. Add the onion and carrot and cook, stirring occasionally, until the onion begins to soften, about 2 minutes. Stir in the ginger and garlic and cook until fragrant, about 1 minute. Stir in the red curry paste and cook for 1 minute, then pour in the coconut milk and add the fish sauce, stirring to combine. Bring to a simmer, then add the bell pepper and broccoli. Reduce the heat to medium, cover, and cook, stirring occasionally, until the broccoli is just shy of tender, about 10 minutes. Add the shrimp, scallops, and mussels and stir to combine. Re-cover and cook until the mussels open, about 5 minutes.

Discard any mussels that haven't opened. Ladle the curry into 4 bowls, garnish with the cilantro, and serve with the lime wedges and, if desired, with the Cauliflower "Rice" (page 156).

Nutritional analysis per serving: *Calories: 503, Fat: 28 g, Saturated Fat: 17 g, Cholesterol: 107 mg, Fiber: 3 g, Protein: 37 g, Carbohydrates: 24 g, Sodium: 1128 mg*

ZUPPA DI PESCE

Serves: 4

Prep time:
30 minutes

Cook time:
45 minutes

Zuppa di pesce is a classic Italian seafood stew with a tomato and wine base. What's essential here is really fresh fish and shellfish, as they will taste best and be most nutritious. I prefer the stew made with a combination of wild-caught firm-textured whitefish, mussels, clams, shrimp, and squid, but use the types of fish and shellfish that are the freshest and most appealing to you.

- 1 (28-ounce) can whole peeled tomatoes
- ¼ cup extra-virgin olive oil
- 1 large yellow onion, roughly chopped
- 4 garlic cloves, minced
- ¼ cup loosely packed fresh parsley leaves, roughly chopped
- 1 teaspoon crushed red pepper flakes
- 1 cup dry white wine
- 1½ pounds cleaned squid tubes, cut into ¼-inch rings, and/or large shell-on shrimp
- 1 pound skinless firm whitefish fillets (such as snapper, cod, haddock, striped bass), cut into 1-inch chunks
- 1 pound mussels and/or clams, scrubbed and debearded (if using mussels)
- sea salt
- ¼ teaspoon freshly ground black pepper

In a blender or food processor, puree the tomatoes with their juice until smooth.

In a Dutch oven or large stockpot, warm the olive oil over medium heat until shimmering. Add the onion and cook, stirring occasionally, until it begins to soften, 3 to 4 minutes. Stir in the garlic and half of the parsley and cook until the garlic is fragrant, about 1 minute. Raise the heat to high, add the red pepper flakes, and pour in the wine. Simmer until the wine is reduced by half, about 3 minutes, then reduce the heat to medium. Pour in the pureed tomatoes and simmer, stirring occasionally, for 5 minutes to allow the flavors to mingle.

Using a large spoon, begin adding the seafood to the pot: if using squid, add it first and cook for 10 minutes. Next, add the shrimp, if using, and the chunked whitefish and cook for 2 minutes. Finally, add the mussels and/or clams, then reduce the heat to low and cook, uncovered, until the mussels and/or clams have opened, about 15 minutes. Season to taste with salt and stir in the black pepper.

Transfer the soup to a warmed tureen, discarding any mussels and/or clams that failed to open, and sprinkle with the remaining parsley. Bring the tureen to the table along with a ladle and serve.

Nutritional analysis per serving: *Calories: 571, Fat: 22 g, Saturated Fat: 2 g, Cholesterol: 398 mg, Fiber: 2 g, Protein: 61 g, Carbohydrates: 21 g, Sodium: 177 mg*

12

Poultry

SHREDDED CHICKEN

Serves: 4

Prep time:
5 minutes

Cook time:
1½ hours,
plus cooling

Making shredded, or "pulled," chicken might seem like a lot of work, but it's easier than you might think. Gently simmering a whole chicken for 1½ hours breaks down the meat into tender pieces that flake off the bones with ease. Use the shredded meat in salads, toss it with Gingery Barbecue Sauce (page 277), or use it as a topping for Savory Coconut Pancakes (page 149).

- 1 (3- to 4-pound) whole chicken
- 1 small yellow onion, roughly chopped
- 3 garlic cloves, cut in half
- 1 tablespoon paprika
- 2 bay leaves
- 2 tablespoons apple cider vinegar

Place all of the ingredients into a large pot and pour in 4 cups filtered water. Cover and bring to a boil over high heat, then reduce the heat to medium and simmer until the chicken breaks apart easily and the meat is very tender, about 1½ hours.

Uncover the pot and allow to stand until the chicken is cool enough to handle. Remove the chicken from the pot; discard the liquid. Using your fingers, pick all the meat off the bones, shredding the large pieces; discard the chicken skin and bones. Use the shredded chicken right away or refrigerate in an airtight container for up to 4 days.

Nutritional analysis per serving (1½ cups): Calories: 589, Fat: 25 g, Saturated Fat: 9 g, Cholesterol: 315 mg, Fiber: 1 g, Protein: 81 g, Carbohydrates: 6 g, Sodium: 264 mg

CHICKEN CUTLETS WITH MIXED GREENS

Serves: 4

Prep time:
30 minutes

Cook time:
10 minutes

Chicken cutlets are extremely versatile. They can be served with a simple side, as they are here; they can be sliced and used as a component in a main-course salad; or they can even be topped with tomato sauce and baked. Chipotle Mayonnaise (page 267) is a delicious dipping sauce for chicken cutlets served on crisp lettuce.

- 2 large boneless, skinless chicken breasts
- ¼ cup coconut flour
- ¼ cup teff flour
- 2 tablespoons potato starch
- ½ teaspoon sea salt, plus more for seasoning
- ½ teaspoon freshly ground black pepper
- 3 large eggs
- 2 tablespoons unsweetened Nut Milk (see page 54)
- ¼ cup Ghee (page 279)
- 8 cups mesclun
- 4 tablespoons extra-virgin olive oil
- 8 cherry tomatoes, cut in half
- 1 lemon, cut into 8 wedges

Place a chicken breast on a cutting board. With a sharp chef's knife held so the flat of the blade is parallel with the board, slice through the thickness of the breast, cutting it into two thin pieces. Repeat with the second chicken breast. Working one at a time, place the pieces between two sheets of parchment paper and gently pound with a meat pounder to an even ½-inch thickness.

In a shallow baking dish, stir together the coconut flour, teff flour, potato starch, ½ teaspoon of salt, and the pepper.

In a second shallow baking dish, whisk together the eggs and nut milk.

One at a time, dredge the chicken cutlets in the flour mixture, shake off the excess, then dip into the egg mixture, coating both sides. Let the excess egg drip off and dredge once again in the flour mixture. Set the coated cutlets on a large plate.

Line a second large plate with paper towels. In a large skillet, warm the ghee over medium-high heat until shimmering. Add the cutlets and cook until golden brown on both sides, 2 to 3 minutes per side. Transfer the cutlets to the prepared plate and season to taste with salt.

Divide the greens among 4 plates and drizzle each portion with 1 tablespoon of the olive oil. Top each portion of greens with 4 cherry tomato halves and place a chicken cutlet and 2 lemon wedges alongside. Serve.

Nutritional analysis per serving: *Calories: 474, Fat: 26 g, Saturated Fat: 7 g, Cholesterol: 237 mg, Fiber: 7 g, Protein: 35 g, Carbohydrates: 26 g, Sodium: 673 mg*

SAUTÉED CHICKEN AND VEGETABLES

Serves: 4

Prep time:
15 minutes

Cook time:
10 minutes

Even though we all live busy lives, we can still cook and eat nutritious, high-quality meals. With this chicken dish that's loaded with healthful veggies, you can get dinner on the table in less than 30 minutes *and* please everyone in the family.

- 2 tablespoons Ghee (page 279)
- 2 large boneless, skinless chicken breasts, cut crosswise into ½-inch strips
- 1 large red onion, thinly sliced
- 1 bunch asparagus, trimmed and cut crosswise into fourths
- 2 large red bell peppers, seeded and sliced into thin strips
- 1 bunch lacinato kale, stemmed and roughly chopped
- juice of 1 lemon
- sea salt
- ½ teaspoon freshly ground black pepper

In a large skillet, warm the ghee over medium-high heat until it begins to smoke. Add the chicken breasts and sauté until cooked halfway through, about 3 minutes. Add the onion, asparagus, and bell peppers and cook, stirring frequently, until the vegetables are tender, about 3 more minutes. Stir in the kale and lemon juice, cover, and cook, stirring occasionally, until the kale is wilted and tender, 2 to 3 minutes.

Season to taste with salt, stir in the black pepper, and serve.

Nutritional analysis per serving: *Calories: 263, Fat: 11 g, Saturated Fat: 5 g, Cholesterol: 86 mg, Fiber: 4 g, Protein: 29 g, Carbohydrates: 11 g, Sodium: 650 mg*

CHICKEN AND KELP NOODLE STIR-FRY

Serves: 4

Prep time:
20 minutes

Cook time:
10 minutes

This recipe is great for using up leftover roasted or grilled chicken; slices of left-over steak work well, too. Stir-fries cook very quickly, so make sure you have all your ingredients prepped and ready to go before turning on the burner.

- 2 tablespoons sesame oil
- 4 garlic cloves, minced
- 1 (1-inch) piece ginger, peeled and minced
- 6 large white button mushrooms, thinly sliced
- 2 cups shredded napa cabbage
- 1 red bell pepper, seeded and thinly sliced
- ¼ cup coconut aminos
- 2 tablespoons rice vinegar
- 2 tablespoons Worcestershire sauce
- 8 to 10 ounces cooked boneless, skinless chicken breast, thinly sliced
- 1 (1-pound) package kelp noodles, cut into 4-inch sections, soaked in warm water for 10 minutes, then drained
- ½ cup loosely packed cilantro leaves, roughly chopped
- 4 scallions, green parts only, thinly sliced
- ¼ cup roasted unsalted cashews, roughly chopped

In a large skillet, warm the sesame oil over high heat until shimmering. Add the garlic and ginger and cook, stirring constantly, until fragrant, about 1 minute. Add the mushrooms, toss a few times, then add the cabbage and bell pepper. Cook, tossing frequently, until the vegetables have softened, 2 to 3 minutes. Pour in the coconut aminos, vinegar, and Worcestershire sauce, stirring well after each addition. Add the chicken, stir to combine, and cook just until the chicken is warmed through, 1 to 2 minutes. Add the kelp noodles and toss well. Stir in the cilantro and scallion greens.

Divide the stir-fry among 4 plates, sprinkle with the cashews, and serve.

Nutritional analysis per serving: *Calories: 287, Fat: 12 g, Saturated Fat: 2 g, Cholesterol: 508 mg, Fiber: 0 g, Protein: 14 g, Carbohydrates: 1 g, Sodium: 426 mg*

Slow-Cooked Chicken with Thai Flavors

Serves: 4

Prep time:
10 minutes

Cook time:
3 hours
(unattended)

In this recipe, flavorful ingredients and a simple cooking method combine to create an amazingly tasty Thai-influenced chicken dish. Serve this dish with Cauliflower "Rice" with Scallions (page 156).

- 1 (3- to 4-pound) whole chicken
- 1 lime, sliced into thin slices
- 1 dried red chile
- 1 (2-inch) piece ginger, peeled and minced
- 5 garlic cloves, minced
- 2 tablespoons finely chopped fresh lemongrass
- 2 teaspoons ground coriander
- 1 (13.5-ounce) can full-fat coconut milk
- 2 tablespoons fish sauce
- ½ bunch cilantro, stemmed and roughly chopped

Preheat the oven to 325°F.

Place the chicken in a 4-quart Dutch oven and add the lime slices, chile, ginger, garlic, lemongrass, coriander, coconut milk, and fish sauce. Cover the pot, place it in the oven, and cook, occasionally spooning the cooking liquid over the chicken, until the chicken is completely tender, about 3 hours.

Carefully remove the chicken from the pot and allow to cool slightly. Pull the meat into large shreds and place in a bowl; discard the skin and bones. Remove and discard the lime, and place the contents of the pot in a blender. Blend on high speed until well pureed, about 45 seconds. Pour the puree through a fine-mesh strainer set over the bowl containing the chicken. Stir the puree into the chicken until well combined. Sprinkle with the cilantro and serve.

Nutritional analysis per serving: Calories: 588, Fat: 58 g, Saturated Fat: 31 g, Cholesterol: 44 mg, Fiber: 4 g, Protein: 19 g, Carbohydrates: 34 g, Sodium: 887 mg

CHICKEN CACCIATORE

Serves: 4

Prep time:
10 minutes

Cook time:
1 hour

This rustic Italian dish is one of my favorites. It can be on the dinner table in 60 minutes, but with such big, bold flavors, it tastes like it's been simmering for hours.

- 8 chicken drumsticks
- ½ teaspoon sea salt
- ½ teaspoon freshly ground black pepper
- 2 tablespoons Ghee (page 279)
- 1 small yellow onion, thinly sliced
- 1 large carrot, scrubbed and finely diced
- 1 red bell pepper, seeded and thinly sliced
- 3 garlic cloves, minced
- 1 teaspoon finely chopped fresh rosemary
- 1 bay leaf
- ½ cup white wine
- 1 (28-ounce) can whole peeled tomatoes, crushed by hand
- ½ cup Kalamata olives, pitted and roughly chopped
- 2 tablespoons drained capers, roughly chopped
- ½ cup loosely packed fresh parsley leaves, roughly chopped

Season the drumsticks with the salt and pepper.

In a 12-inch skillet, warm the ghee over medium-high heat until shimmering. Add the drumsticks to the pan and cook, turning occasionally, until browned on all sides, 5 to 6 minutes total. Transfer the chicken to a large plate and add the onion, carrot, and bell pepper to the pan. Cook, stirring occasionally, until the vegetables are lightly browned, about 5 minutes. Stir in the garlic and rosemary, then add the bay leaf and wine. Using a wooden spoon, scrape up the browned bits on the bottom of the pan, then simmer until the liquid is reduced by about half, about 3 minutes. Stir in the tomatoes with their juice and return the drumsticks to the pan. Cover, reduce the heat to medium, and simmer until the chicken is tender and opaque throughout, about 30 minutes.

Stir in the olives, capers, and parsley. Place 2 drumsticks on each of 4 plates, generously spoon sauce over the chicken, and serve.

Nutritional analysis per serving: Calories: 315, Fat: 15 g, Saturated Fat: 6 g, Cholesterol: 56 mg, Fiber: 5 g, Protein: 19 g, Carbohydrates: 21 g, Sodium: 792 mg

Braised Chicken Thighs with Tomatillos

The dark-meat sections (thighs and drumsticks) of poultry are rich and flavorful, but they can be a bit tough, especially if they come from good-quality free-range birds. Braising is a gentle cooking technique that tenderizes tough cuts, and it also results in a flavorful sauce to accompany the meat. Here, cumin-seasoned chicken thighs are braised with tomatillos, onion, and jalapeño for a tasty dish with Mexican flair.

Serves: 4

Prep time: 15 minutes

Cook time: 45 minutes

- 8 boneless, skin-on chicken thighs
- 2 teaspoons ground cumin
- ¾ teaspoon sea salt
- ½ teaspoon freshly ground black pepper
- 1 tablespoon avocado oil
- 1 large yellow onion, cut into ¼-inch dice
- 3 garlic cloves, finely chopped
- 6 tomatillos, husked and quartered
- 1 jalapeño, thinly sliced
- 2 cups chicken stock
- ½ cup Chipotle Mayonnaise (page 267)
- grated zest and juice of 1 lime
- ¼ cup fresh cilantro leaves, roughly chopped
- 1 large avocado, pitted, peeled, and cut into chunks

Season the chicken thighs with the cumin, salt, and pepper.

In a Dutch oven, warm the avocado oil over medium-high heat until shimmering. Place the chicken thighs skin side down in a single layer in the pot and cook until browned, 3 to 4 minutes. Flip the thighs and cook until the second sides are lightly browned, about 2 minutes. Add the onion and garlic and cook, stirring occasionally, until the onion begins to soften, 1 to 2 minutes. Add the tomatillos, jalapeño slices, and chicken stock, and bring to a boil. Reduce the heat to medium, cover, and simmer until the chicken is tender and opaque throughout, about 30 minutes.

While the chicken cooks, in a small bowl, stir together the chipotle mayonnaise, lime zest and juice, and cilantro.

Divide the chicken and sauce among 4 plates. Top each portion with a spoonful of the chipotle mayonnaise mixture and the avocado chunks and serve.

Nutritional analysis per serving: *Calories: 627, Fat: 45 g, Saturated Fat: 10 g, Cholesterol: 164 mg, Fiber: 4 g, Protein: 39 g, Carbohydrates: 21 g, Sodium: 746 mg*

Mustard-Orange Baked Chicken Legs with Wilted Radicchio

Serves: 4

Prep time:
15 minutes

Cook time:
45 minutes

PEGAN DIET

Slightly bitter and spicy radicchio is a good source of antioxidants. Here it is paired with baked chicken to create a crowd-pleasing recipe. The combination of piquant mustard and bright, sweet orange adds bold flavor to the rich dark-meat parts of the chicken.

- 4 skin-on chicken legs, divided at the joint into thighs and drumsticks
- 2 navel oranges, 1 juiced, 1 cut into 8 wedges
- 2 teaspoons paprika
- 1 teaspoon dry mustard
- 4 tablespoons extra-virgin olive oil
- 2 teaspoons red wine vinegar
- 2 teaspoons Dijon mustard
- 2 large heads radicchio, cored and shredded
- 1 tablespoon fresh lemon juice
- ½ teaspoon sea salt
- 3 sprigs thyme, leaves only, finely chopped

Preheat the oven to 375°F.

Place the chicken parts in a large bowl and add the orange juice and wedges, paprika, dry mustard, 2 tablespoons of the olive oil, the vinegar, and the Dijon mustard. Toss until well combined and the chicken is evenly coated. Arrange the chicken pieces and orange wedges in a single layer on a baking sheet. Bake for 30 minutes, flip the chicken pieces, and continue to bake until tender and opaque throughout, about 15 more minutes.

During the last 5 minutes of baking the chicken, in a large skillet, warm the remaining 2 tablespoons olive oil over medium-high heat until shimmering. Add the radicchio and cook, stirring frequently, until completely wilted, about 3 minutes. Stir in the lemon juice and salt.

Scatter the radicchio on a platter, then arrange the chicken pieces and orange wedges on top. Sprinkle with the thyme and serve.

Nutritional analysis per serving: Calories: 453, Fat: 21 g, Saturated Fat: 4 g, Cholesterol: 122 mg, Fiber: 2 g, Protein: 24 g, Carbohydrates: 10 g, Sodium: 435 mg

CHICKEN, ASPARAGUS, AND TOMATO WITH BROWN RICE

PEGAN DIET

After a long week of work or travel, I love to cook up a warm and comforting meal like this dish. It contains ingredients that provide deep nourishment, but if you're on the twenty-one-day *Eat Fat, Get Thin* Plan, substitute Cauliflower "Rice" (see page 156) for the brown rice.

Serves: 4

Prep time: 15 minutes

Cook time: 20 minutes

- 1 cup long-grain brown rice
- 2¼ cups chicken stock
- 2 tablespoons Ghee (page 279)
- 3 garlic cloves, crushed
- 2 large boneless, skinless chicken breasts, cut crosswise into ½-inch-thick strips
- 2 bunches asparagus, trimmed and cut into thirds
- 1 large tomato, roughly chopped
- ½ cup tomato puree
- 1 cup chicken stock or filtered water
- 2 sprigs thyme, leaves only, finely chopped
- ½ teaspoon sea salt
- ½ teaspoon freshly ground black pepper
- 2 tablespoons unsalted, grass-fed butter

In a saucepan, combine the rice and chicken stock. Cover and bring to a boil over high heat, then reduce the heat to medium and simmer until all the water is absorbed, about 15 minutes. Remove the pan from the heat and allow to stand, covered, for 5 minutes.

While the rice cooks, in a large skillet, warm the ghee over medium–high heat until melted. Add the garlic and cook, stirring frequently, until the garlic just starts to brown, about 2 minutes. Add the chicken, scattering the slices in a single layer, and cook without stirring; initially the slices will stick to the pan, but after about 3 minutes, when nearly halfway cooked, they will release easily. At this point, add the asparagus, toss to combine, then add the tomato, tomato puree, and chicken stock. Stir to combine, cover the pan, and simmer until the chicken is cooked through and the asparagus is tender, about 3 minutes. Stir in the thyme, salt, and pepper, then stir in the butter until incorporated.

Divide the rice among 4 bowls. Spoon the chicken mixture over the rice and serve.

Nutritional analysis per serving: Calories: 422, Fat: 19 g, Saturated Fat: 10 g, Cholesterol: 106 mg, Fiber: 5 g, Protein: 36 g, Carbohydrates: 28 g, Sodium: 1781 mg

CHICKEN WITH SOFRITO AND SPINACH

Sofrito, a flavorful combination of slow-cooked, finely chopped aromatic vegetables, is a perfect seasoning for a mild-tasting chicken. Spinach boosts the nutrition of this already hearty and healthful dish.

Serves: 4

Prep time: 15 minutes

Cook time: 1 hour

- 4 skin-on chicken legs
- 1 teaspoon sea salt
- 1 tablespoon Ghee (page 279) or lard
- 1 cup dry white wine
- 1 cup Dr. Hyman's Veggie-Bone Broth (page 128)
- 1 cup Sofrito (page 284)
- 12 cups baby spinach

Preheat the oven to 350°F.

Season the chicken legs with the salt. In a large ovenproof skillet, warm the ghee over medium-high heat until shimmering. Place the chicken skin side down in the pan and cook until browned, 4 to 5 minutes. Flip the legs and cook until the second sides are lightly browned, about 2 minutes. Transfer to a large plate. Pour the wine into the pan and simmer until reduced by about half. Return the chicken legs, skin side up, to the pan. Pour in the bone broth, then place ¼ cup sofrito on top of each leg and use a spoon to spread it over the entire surface. Cover the pan, then place it in the oven and bake until the chicken is tender and opaque throughout, about 45 minutes.

Remove the pan from the oven. Uncover and stir in the spinach. Re-cover and allow to stand until the spinach is wilted, about 2 minutes.

Transfer 1 chicken leg, along with spinach and sauce, to each of 4 plates. Serve.

Nutritional analysis per serving: *Calories: 305, Fat: 17 g, Saturated Fat: 5 g, Cholesterol: 125 mg, Fiber: 3 g, Protein: 28 g, Carbohydrates: 9 g, Sodium: 748 mg*

ZA'ATAR ROASTED CHICKEN

Serves: 4

Prep time:
5 minutes

Cook time:
1¼ hours

Za'atar is a Middle Eastern seasoning blend that typically includes sesame seeds, sumac, and the dried herb called *za'atar*. It is often sprinkled onto flatbreads, but the flavors also work well with chicken. Look for *za'atar* in well-stocked grocery stores or in Middle Eastern markets, or purchase it at online spice shops.

- 4 tablespoons salted, grass-fed butter
- 2 tablespoons za'atar
- 1 (3- to 4-pound) whole chicken
- 1 lemon, cut into 4 wedges

Preheat the oven to 425°F.

In a small saucepan, warm the butter and za'atar over medium heat until the butter is melted.

Place the chicken in a baking dish. Loosen the skin over the breasts and brush some of the za'atar butter under the skin, directly onto the meat, then brush the remaining butter all over the exterior.

Roast the chicken for 20 minutes, then reduce the oven temperature to 325°F and continue to roast until the meat is opaque throughout and the internal temperature of the thickest part of the breast is 165°F on an instant-read thermometer, 40 to 45 more minutes.

Allow the chicken to rest for 5 minutes, then carve and serve with the lemon wedges.

Nutritional analysis per serving: Calories: 677, Fat: 37 g, Saturated Fat: 16 g, Cholesterol: 346 mg, Fiber: 1 g, Protein: 81 g, Carbohydrates: 2 g, Sodium: 494 mg

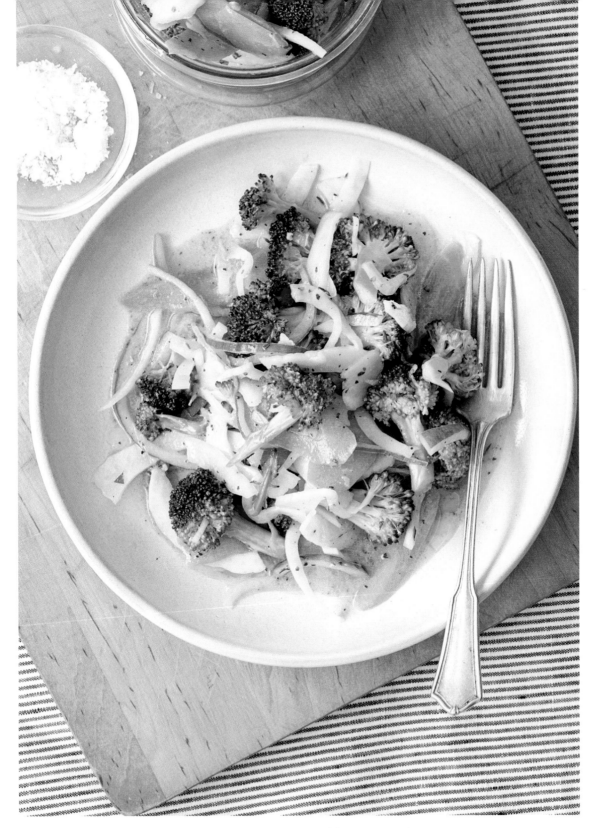

Italian Marinated Vegetables (page 152)

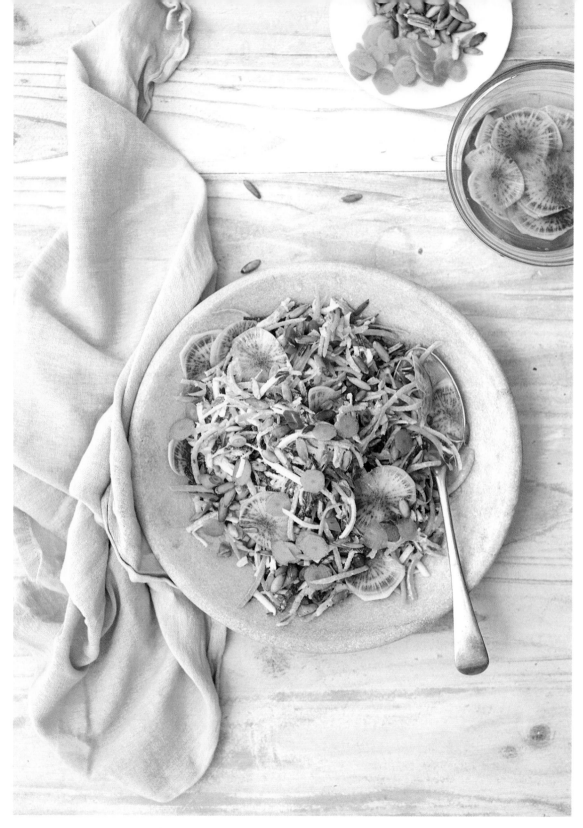

Confetti Vegetable Slaw with Tahini Dressing (page 153)

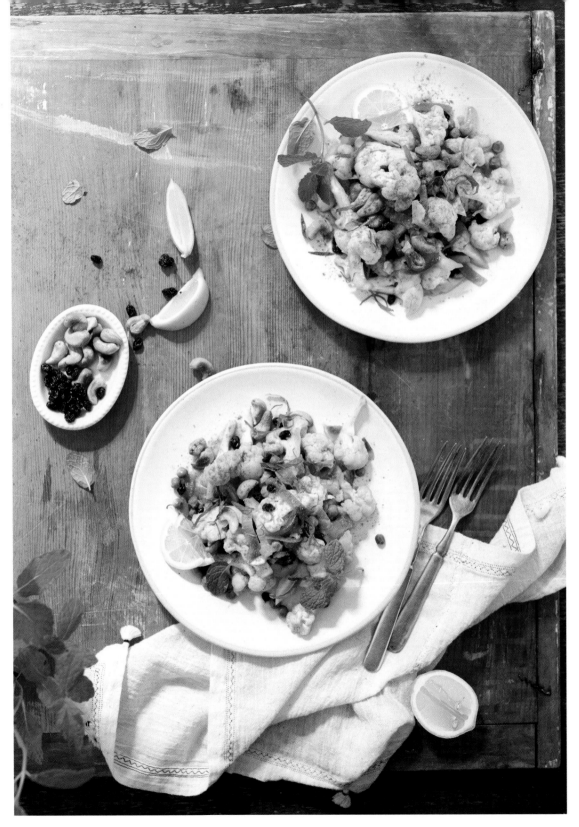

Curried Cauliflower with Peas and Mint (page 157)

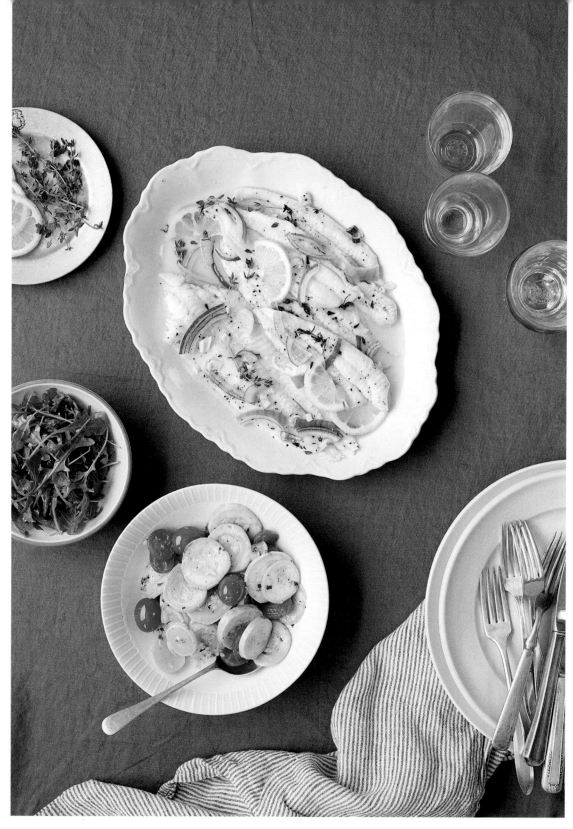

Lemon-Baked Sole with Stewed Summer Squash (page 176)

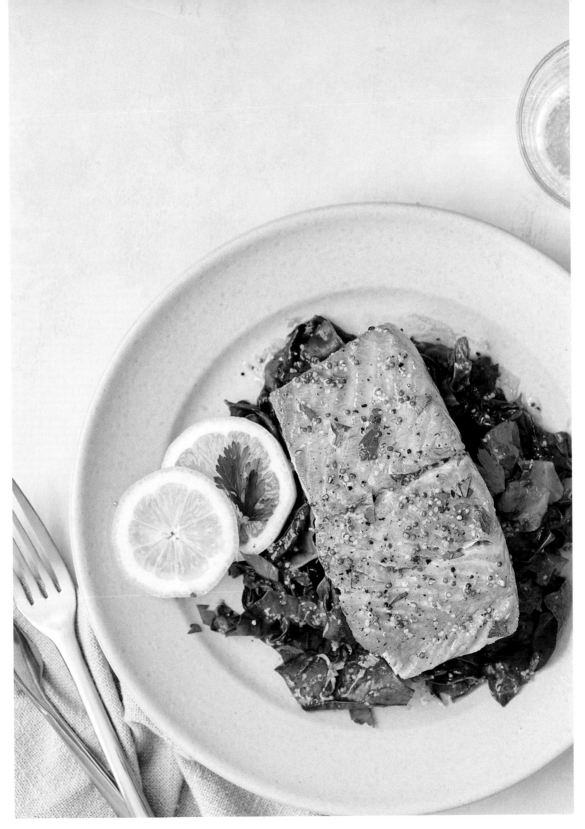

Arctic Char with Swiss Chard and Mustard Vinaigrette (page 182)

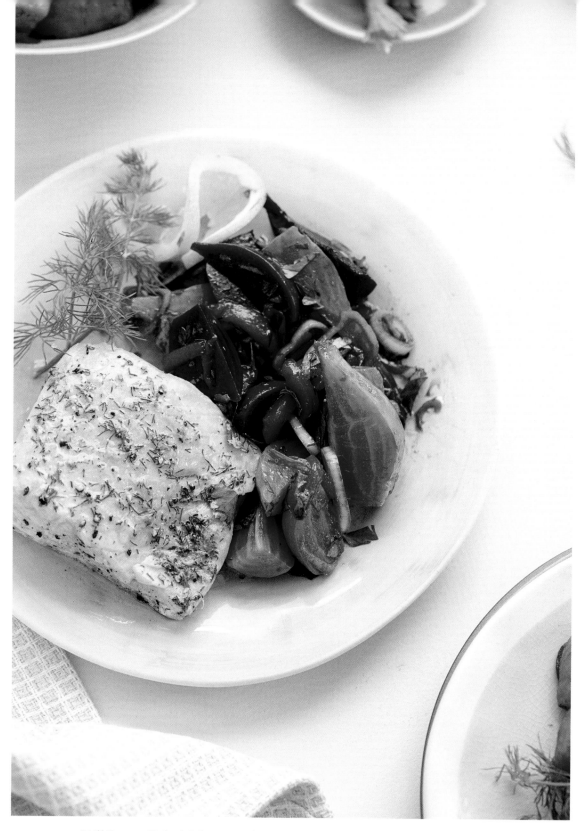

Dill Butter–Baked Salmon with Beet and Roasted Pepper Salad (page 184)

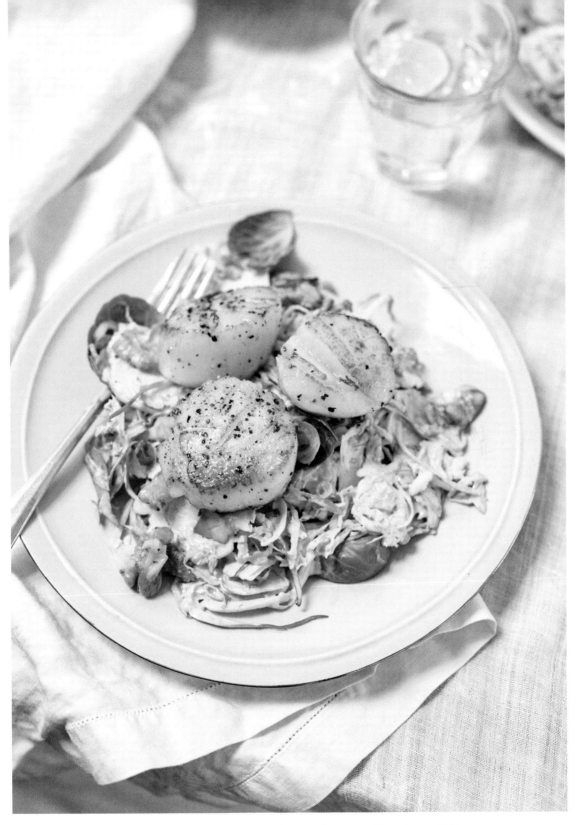

Seared Scallops with Curried Brussels Sprout Slaw (page 193)

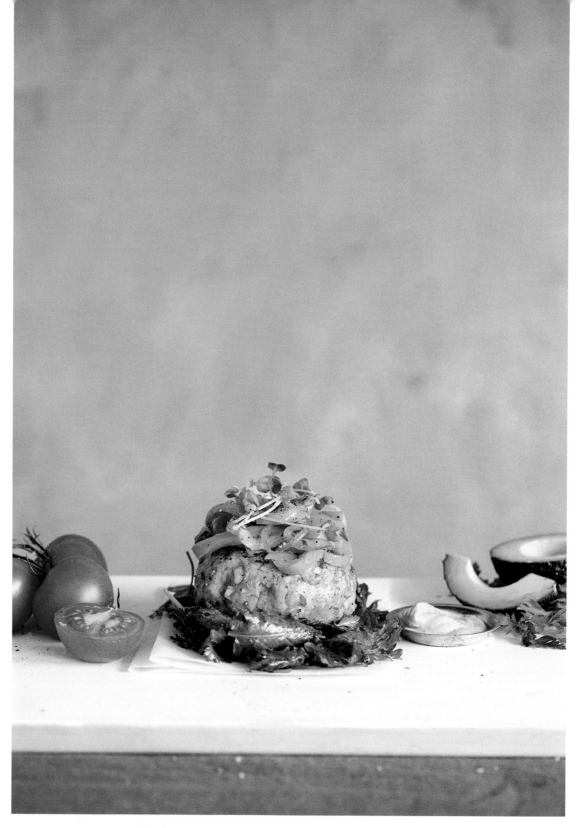

Turkey Burgers with Peppers and Onions (page 220)

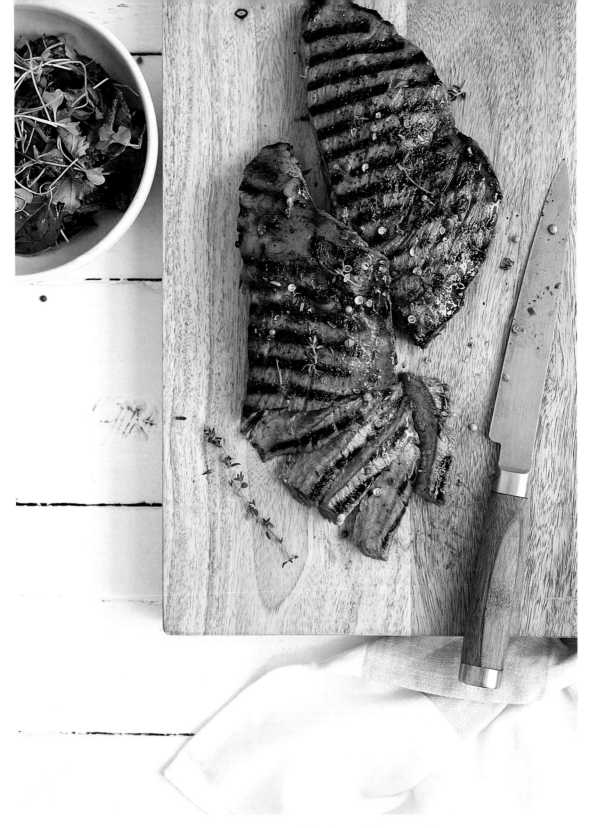

Grilled Miso–Marinated Flank Steak (page 229)

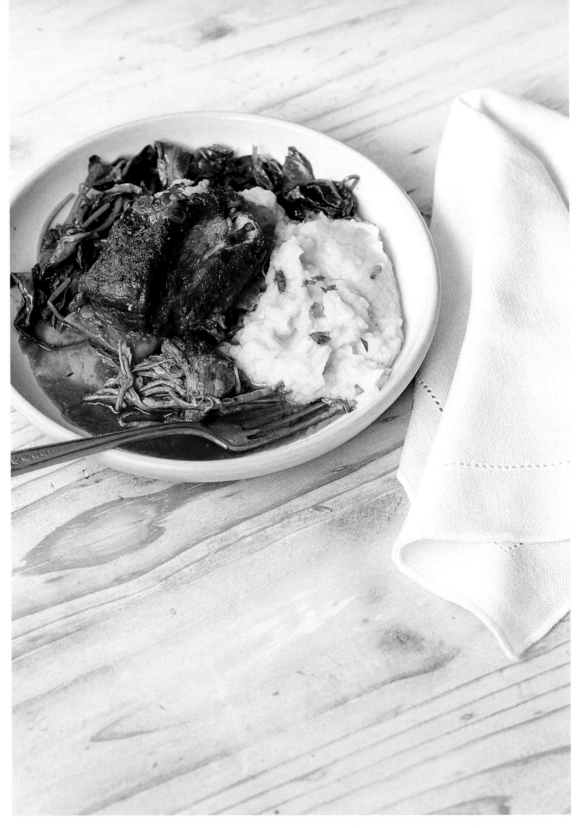

Braised Short Ribs with Fennel Seed and Cider Vinegar (page 239)

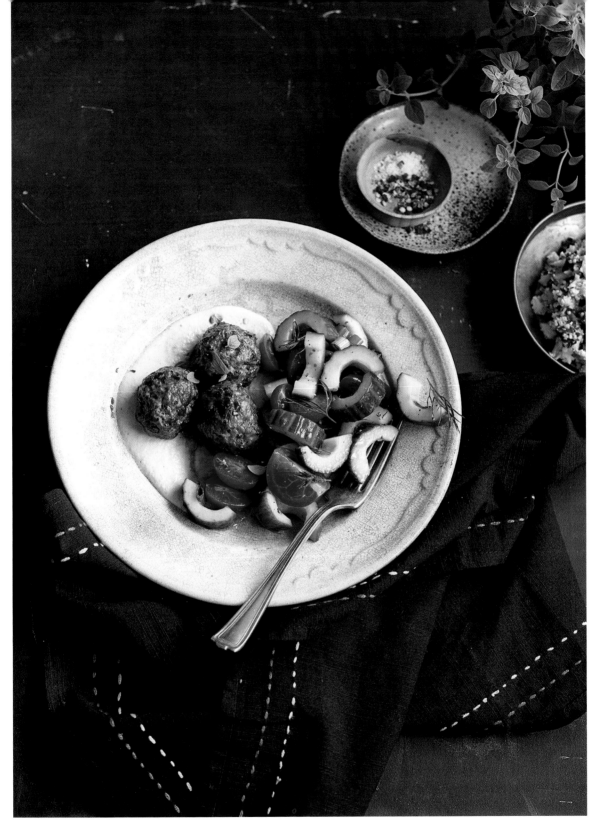

Lamb Meatballs with Tomato–Cucumber Salad and Cashew "Yogurt" (page 245)

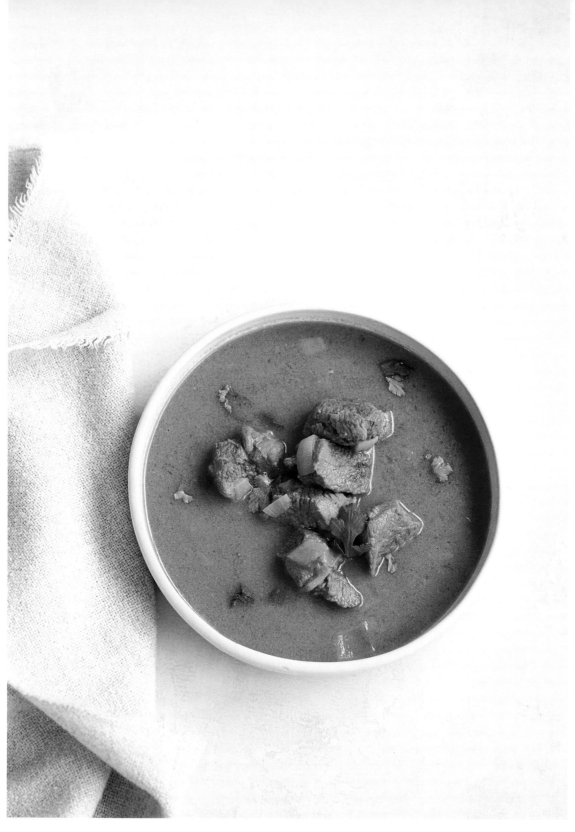

Caribbean Lamb Stew (page 247)

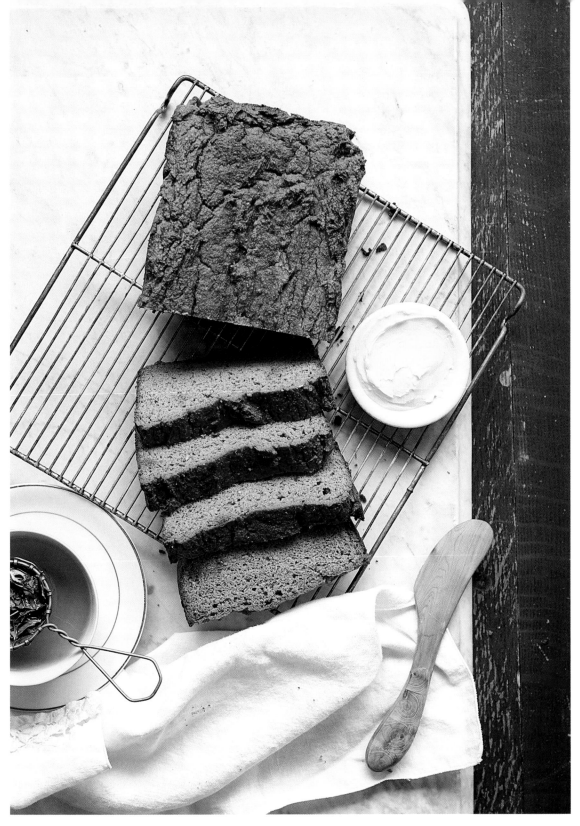

Spiced Sweet Potato Quick Bread (page 251)

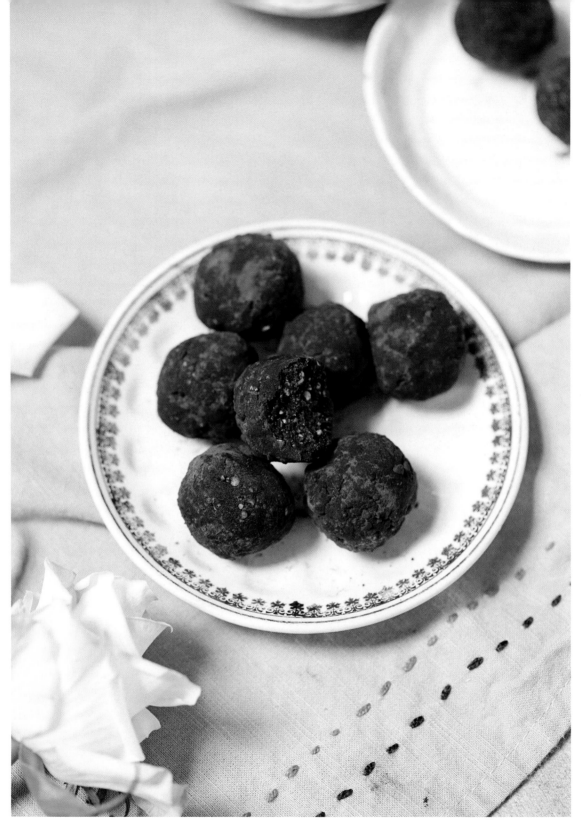

Chocolate Truffles (page 258)

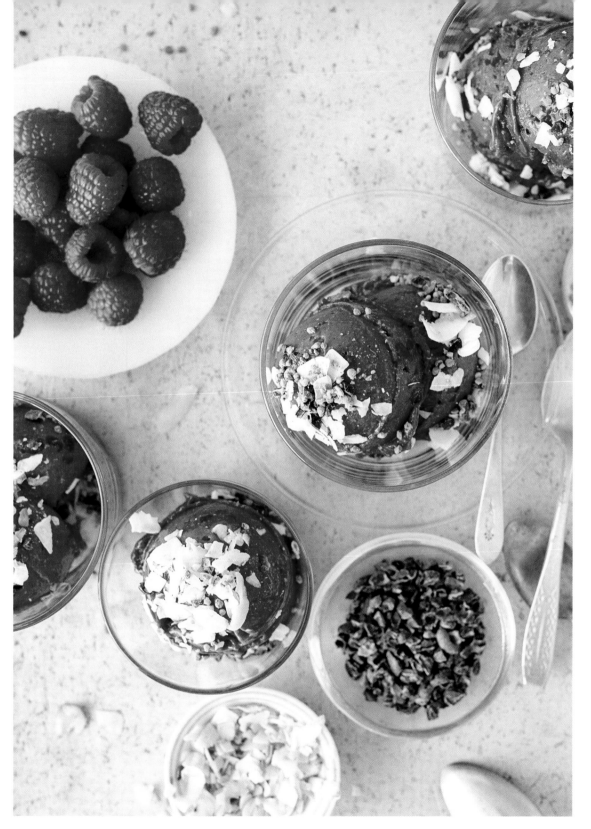

Raspberry-Coconut Ice Cream (page 262)

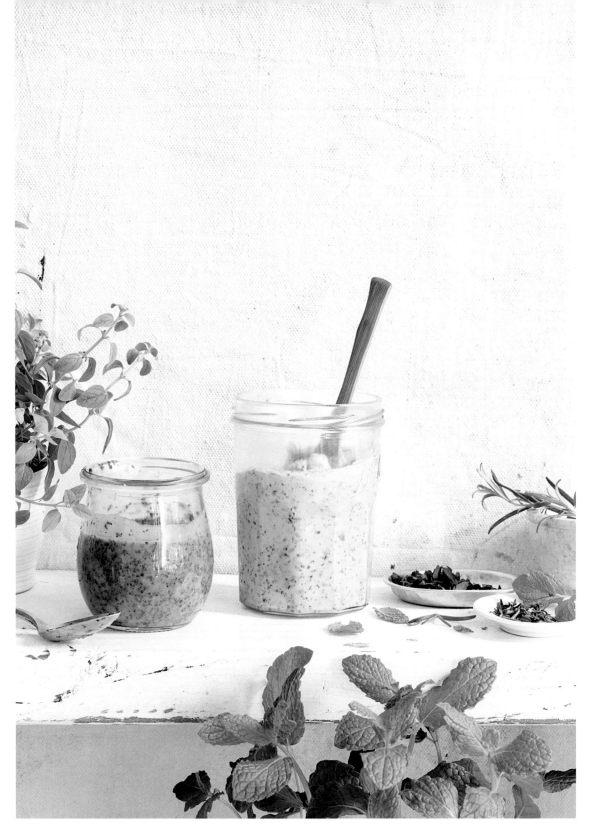

Chimichurri (page 272) and Herbed Compound Butter (page 280)

GRILLED CHICKEN BREASTS WITH SAMBAL

Sambal, a fiery chile paste, is a staple of Indonesian and Malaysian cuisine. Here, a simple homemade sambal is used as a basting sauce for grilled chicken breasts. Sambal can also be used as a condiment, and it keeps in an airtight container in the refrigerator for a few days, so if you like spicy foods, I suggest making a double batch.

- 1 tablespoon coconut oil
- 3 garlic cloves, thinly sliced
- 3 large scallions, thinly sliced
- 10 fresh or dried Thai red chiles, stems removed, seeds discarded if sensitive to spice
- 1 large tomato, roughly chopped
- 1 tablespoon fish sauce
- grated zest and juice of 1 lime
- 4 (6-ounce) boneless, skin-on chicken breasts
- 2 tablespoons extra-virgin olive oil, plus more for the grill grate
- ½ teaspoon sea salt

Serves: 4

Prep time: 20 minutes

Cook time: 30 minutes

To make the sambal, in a 10-inch skillet, warm the coconut oil over medium-high heat until melted. Add the garlic and scallions and cook, stirring occasionally, until golden brown, 3 minutes. Add the chiles, tomato, fish sauce, and lime zest and juice and cook, stirring occasionally, until the tomato begins to break down and its juice evaporates, about 10 minutes. Transfer the mixture to a blender and puree on high speed until smooth. Scoop the sambal into a small bowl and set aside. (The sambal can be refrigerated in an airtight container for up to 5 days.)

Build a medium fire in a charcoal grill or preheat a gas grill to medium.

Coat the chicken breasts with the olive oil and season with the salt. Scrape the grill grate clean and lightly grease it with olive oil. Place the chicken breasts skin side down on the grate and cook until the skin is browned and releases from the grate, about 5 minutes. Flip the breasts, then use a pastry brush to spread sambal on each of the chicken breasts.

Continue to cook, basting once more with the remaining sambal, until the chicken is firm and opaque throughout, 3 to 4 more minutes. Transfer the breasts skin side up to a cutting board and allow them to rest for a few minutes.

Slice the chicken breasts against the grain and serve.

Nutritional analysis per serving: *Calories: 360, Fat: 22 g, Saturated Fat: 7 g, Cholesterol: 63 mg, Fiber: 2 g, Protein: 29 g, Carbohydrates: 12 g, Sodium: 725 mg*

SAUTÉED CHICKEN HEARTS WITH GARLIC AND ROSEMARY

Serves: 4

Prep time:
5 minutes

Cook time:
5 minutes

Often overlooked, chicken hearts are some of the most nutrient-dense parts of the bird. They're a great source of protein, B vitamins, zinc, and iron. If you've never tried chicken hearts, give this simple recipe a go. You'll be surprised by how delicious and satisfying they are.

- 2 tablespoons Ghee (page 279)
- 4 large garlic cloves, thinly sliced
- 1 pound chicken hearts, rinsed and patted dry
- 1 teaspoon minced fresh rosemary
- ½ teaspoon sea salt
- juice of ½ lemon

In a large skillet, warm the ghee over medium-high heat until shimmering. Add the garlic and cook, stirring occasionally, until lightly browned, about 2 minutes. Add the chicken hearts and cook, tossing continuously, until firm, about 4 minutes. Stir in the rosemary and salt, squeeze in some juice from the lemon half, and serve.

Nutritional analysis per serving: *Calories: 248, Fat: 18 g, Saturated Fat: 8 g, Cholesterol: 154 mg, Fiber: 0 g, Protein: 18 g, Carbohydrates: 3 g, Sodium: 645 mg*

TURKEY BURGERS WITH PEPPERS AND ONIONS

Serves: 4

Prep time:
15 minutes

Cook time:
20 minutes

Turkey is a lean, neutral-flavored protein that pairs well with just about any type of seasoning. In this simple recipe, ground turkey meets curry powder, which boasts anti-inflammatory properties because of the spices it contains.

- 1 pound ground turkey
- 1 small onion, minced, plus 1 large onion, thinly sliced
- 1 celery rib, minced
- 2 tablespoons curry powder
- 1 large egg, beaten
- 1 tablespoon coconut flour
- 1 teaspoon sea salt
- 4 tablespoons coconut oil
- 2 bell peppers, seeded and thinly sliced
- ½ teaspoon freshly ground black pepper
- 2 scallions, thinly sliced
- 2 tablespoons chopped fresh parsley

In a bowl, combine the ground turkey, minced onion, celery, curry powder, egg, coconut flour, and ½ teaspoon of salt. Mix until thoroughly combined. Divide the mixture into 4 portions and shape each into a 3-inch patty.

In a large nonstick skillet, warm 2 tablespoons of the coconut oil over medium heat until shimmering. Add the patties and cook, flipping them once, until browned and firm and cooked through, about 15 minutes total.

While the burgers cook, in a large skillet, warm the remaining 2 tablespoons coconut oil over medium heat until shimmering. Add the sliced onion and bell peppers and cook, stirring occasionally, until softened, about 10 minutes. Stir in the remaining salt and the pepper, scallions, and parsley.

Place 1 burger on each of 4 plates. Top the patties with the onion and pepper mixture, dividing it evenly, and serve. Pairs nicely with a small bed of greens and avocado (optional).

Nutritional analysis per serving: *Calories: 417, Fat: 23 g, Saturated Fat: 10 g, Cholesterol: 152 mg, Fiber: 6 g, Protein: 36 g, Carbohydrates: 19 g, Sodium: 693 mg*

SLOW-COOKED DUCK LEGS WITH SPICED CHERRY SAUCE AND WHITE BEAN PUREE

Serves: 4

Prep time:
10 minutes

Cook time:
1¾ hours

PEGAN DIET

Duck may be a bit pricey, but it's a great source of monounsaturated fat, so it's worth the indulgence. The deep, rich flavor of duck pairs well with fruits and spices—I particularly like this combination of duck with cherries and warm spices. If you omit the white bean puree, you can enjoy this dish during the twenty-one-day plan.

- 4 duck legs
- ½ teaspoon sea salt
- ¼ teaspoon freshly ground black pepper
- 1 tablespoon Ghee (page 279)
- 1 cup fresh or thawed frozen sweet cherries, pitted
- 4 cups Dr. Hyman's Veggie-Bone Broth (page 128)
- 2 whole star anise
- 5 cardamom pods
- 1 vanilla bean, cut in half lengthwise
- White Bean Puree with Rosemary (page 150), warmed

Preheat the oven to 325°F.

Season the duck legs with the salt and pepper. In a large Dutch oven, warm the ghee over medium-high heat until melted. Place the duck legs skin side down in the pot and cook until lightly browned and some of the fat has rendered, 4 to 5 minutes. Pour off the fat in the pot, then add the cherries, bone broth, star anise, cardamom, and vanilla bean. Bring to a boil, cover, and transfer the pot to the oven. Cook until the meat is tender and the cooking liquid is slightly reduced, about 1½ hours.

Transfer the duck legs to a plate and cover with aluminum foil to keep warm. Pour the cooking liquid through a fine-mesh sieve set over a small saucepan; discard the solids in the sieve. Set the pan over low heat and bring the cooking liquid to a simmer.

Divide the bean puree among 4 plates and place a duck leg on top. Spoon a few tablespoons of the cooking liquid over each duck leg and serve.

Nutritional analysis per serving: *Calories: 306, Fat: 15 g, Saturated Fat: 5 g, Cholesterol: 105 mg, Fiber: 2 g, Protein: 27 g, Carbohydrates: 15 g, Sodium: 932 mg*

13

Beef and Lamb

Ground Beef and Butternut Sauté

I love the balance of sweet, spicy, and herbal in this quick-cooking one-pot dish. Although this recipe calls for butternut squash, you can substitute any winter squash or root vegetable you prefer or have on hand.

- 2 tablespoons Ghee (page 279)
- 1 large onion, finely diced
- 1 pound grass-fed ground beef
- 2 teaspoons paprika
- ¾ teaspoon sea salt
- ½ small butternut squash, peeled, seeded, and shredded (about 4 cups)
- 2 (4-inch) sprigs rosemary, leaves only, finely chopped

In a large skillet, warm the ghee over medium-high heat until melted. Add the onion and cook, stirring occasionally, until softened, 3 to 4 minutes. Add the beef and cook, using a spatula to break up the meat and combine it with the onion, until the beef is no longer pink, 3 to 4 minutes. Add the paprika and salt and cook, stirring occasionally, for 5 minutes. Add the shredded butternut squash and continue to cook, stirring occasionally, until the squash is tender and the beef is thoroughly cooked, about 2 minutes. Stir in the rosemary.

Divide the mixture among 4 plates and serve.

Nutritional analysis per serving: *Calories: 320, Fat: 13 g, Saturated Fat: 6 g, Cholesterol: 60 mg, Fiber: 6 g, Protein: 25 g, Carbohydrates: 31 g, Sodium: 518 mg*

"Spaghetti" and Meatballs with Tomato Sauce

Serves: 4

Prep time:
15 minutes

Cook time:
30 minutes

This is my kind of Sunday supper to enjoy with the family. Spaghetti squash baked until tender and separated into noodle-like strands is a perfect gluten-free replacement for regular pasta. To help simplify cooking, the squash can be cooked the day before and reheated on the stove top while the meatballs simmer in the sauce.

- 2 tablespoons extra-virgin olive oil
- 1 large spaghetti squash, halved lengthwise and seeded
- 1 pound grass-fed ground beef
- 1 small yellow onion, minced
- 1 teaspoon garlic powder
- ½ cup fresh parsley leaves, roughly chopped
- 1 teaspoon sea salt
- ½ teaspoon freshly ground black pepper
- 2 teaspoons fennel seeds, coarsely ground in a spice grinder
- 1 teaspoon crushed red pepper flakes
- 1½ tablespoons chia seeds, ground in a spice grinder
- 2 tablespoons unsalted, grass-fed butter, at room temperature
- 4 garlic cloves, thinly sliced
- 1 (28-ounce) can fire-roasted whole tomatoes, roughly chopped

Preheat the oven to 350°F.

Drizzle 1 tablespoon of the olive oil onto a baking sheet. Place the squash halves cut side down on the baking sheet and bake until the squash is tender, about 25 minutes.

While the squash bakes, in a bowl, combine the beef, onion, garlic powder, parsley, salt, black pepper, fennel seeds, pepper flakes, and chia seeds. Mix until thoroughly combined. Using your hands, form the mixture into 12 evenly sized meatballs and set aside.

When the squash is done, remove the baking sheet from the oven, carefully flip over the squash halves, and let stand until cool enough to handle.

Using a spoon, scrape the squash flesh from the skin, separating it into spaghetti-like strands, and transfer it to a saucepan. Add the butter and toss until the squash is well coated. Cover to keep warm on low heat until ready to serve.

In a skillet, warm the remaining 1 tablespoon olive oil over medium heat until shimmering. Add the sliced garlic and cook, stirring occasionally, until lightly browned, about 2 minutes. Stir in the tomatoes with their juice, cover, and cook for 5 minutes. Add the meatballs, re-cover, and continue to simmer, stirring occasionally, until the meatballs are firm, about 20 minutes.

Divide the spaghetti squash among 4 plates. Top each portion with meatballs and several spoonfuls of sauce and serve.

Nutritional analysis per serving: Calories: 768, Fat: 20 g, Saturated Fat: 7 g, Cholesterol: 75 mg, Fiber: 10 g, Protein: 44 g, Carbohydrates: 115 g, Sodium: 963 mg

MEATLOAF WITH ITALIAN SEASONINGS

Serves: 4

Prep time:
15 minutes

Cook time:
30 minutes

PEGAN DIET

Whenever I can, I spend a little extra time in the kitchen on Sundays to prep for the week ahead. Dishes like meatloaf are fantastic because they can be cooked in advance and eaten over the next several days.

- ½ cup almond meal
- 1½ pounds grass-fed ground beef
- 1 large yellow onion, minced
- ¼ cup coconut flour
- ¾ cup Smoky Ketchup (page 276)
- 3 large eggs, lightly beaten
- ½ bunch parsley, stemmed and roughly chopped
- 2 teaspoons dried thyme
- 1 teaspoon dried oregano
- ½ teaspoon freshly ground black pepper
- 1 tablespoon extra-virgin olive oil

Preheat the oven to 350°F.

In a large bowl, combine the almond meal, beef, onion, and coconut flour, ¼ cup of the ketchup, and the eggs, parsley, thyme, oregano, and pepper. Mix until thoroughly combined, but do not overwork the mixture.

Drizzle the olive oil into the bottom of a 9- by 13-inch baking dish. Transfer the beef mixture to the baking dish and use your hands to form it into a 4- by 4-inch loaf, about 2 inches high. Evenly spread the remaining ½ cup ketchup over the top of the loaf.

Bake until the internal temperature of the meatloaf reaches 160°F on an instant-read thermometer, about 20 minutes. Remove the meatloaf from the oven and baste it with the drippings in the baking dish. Cut into 1-inch slices and serve.

Nutritional analysis per serving: Calories: 423, Fat: 21 g, Saturated Fat: 7 g, Cholesterol: 195 mg, Fiber: 14 g, Protein: 25 g, Carbohydrates: 34 g, Sodium: 617 mg

GRILLED MISO-MARINATED FLANK STEAK

PEGAN DIET

This marinade infuses the flavors of miso paste and dulse into a lean and usually tough cut of meat. Make sure to slice the steak against the grain to help ensure that it's as tender as can be. Enjoy this with Garlic-Steamed Broccoli Rabe (page 159).

- 1¼ pounds beef flank steak
- 2 tablespoons chickpea miso
- 2 tablespoons dulse flakes
- 2 tablespoons wheat-free tamari
- 2 tablespoons toasted sesame oil
- 1 tablespoon rice vinegar
- 1 tablespoon coriander seeds, coarsely ground in a spice grinder
- 1 bunch scallions, white parts only, thinly sliced
- 1 dried red chile, crushed
- 1 tablespoon grated ginger
- olive oil, for greasing the grill grate (if using a charcoal or gas grill)
- sprigs of thyme, for garnish (optional)

Serves: 4

Prep time: 10 minutes, plus marinating time

Cook time: 10 minutes

Place the flank steak in a glass baking dish just large enough to hold it in a single layer.

In a small bowl, whisk together the miso, dulse flakes, tamari, sesame oil, vinegar, coriander seeds, scallions, chile, and ginger until combined. Pour the mixture over the flank steak, then flip the steak a few times to coat evenly with the marinade. Cover and refrigerate for at least 8 hours or up to 12 hours, flipping the steak once.

Heat a large, well-seasoned stove-top grill pan over medium-high heat. Alternatively, build a medium fire in a charcoal grill or preheat a gas grill to medium; when the grill is hot, scrape the grate clean and lightly grease it with olive oil. Remove the steak from the marinade and cook for 3 to 4 minutes per side for medium-rare (130°F); cook for less or more time depending on your desired degree of doneness. Transfer the steak to a cutting board and let rest for 10 minutes.

Cut the steak against the grain into ½-inch slices and serve, garnished with the thyme, if using.

Nutritional analysis per serving: Calories: 379, Fat: 22 g, Saturated Fat: 6 g, Cholesterol: 94 mg, Fiber: 3 g, Protein: 34 g, Carbohydrates: 9 g, Sodium: 829 mg

GRILLED RED WINE AND ROSEMARY SIRLOIN STEAK WITH MUSHROOMS

Serves: 4

Prep time:
15 minutes, plus
marinating time

Cook time:
30 minutes

I love the combination of beef, rosemary, and mushrooms. Button mushrooms and portobellos are great, but to make the dish more interesting, try some unusual varieties such as oyster, chanterelle, or black trumpet.

- 1 small shallot, thinly sliced
- 2 garlic cloves, minced
- grated zest and juice of 1 lemon
- ½ cup red wine
- 1 (4-inch) sprig rosemary, leaves only, finely chopped
- ½ teaspoon sea salt
- ½ teaspoon freshly ground black pepper
- 2 (8-ounce) beef sirloin steaks
- 1 pound mixed mushrooms (such as button, portobello, cremini, oyster, and shiitake)
- 4 tablespoons extra-virgin olive oil, plus more for the grill grate
- 2 tablespoons fresh oregano leaves, roughly chopped
- 1 large sprig thyme, leaves only, finely chopped

In a glass baking dish, combine the shallot, garlic, lemon zest and juice, wine, rosemary, salt, and pepper and mix until the salt dissolves. Add the steaks and turn to coat with the marinade. Cover and refrigerate for at least 6 hours or up to 12 hours.

Build a medium fire in a charcoal grill or preheat a gas grill to medium. While the grill heats, trim any tough stems off the mushrooms and put the mushrooms in a large bowl. Drizzle with 2 tablespoons of the olive oil, add the oregano and thyme, and toss to combine.

Remove the steaks from the marinade, reserve the marinade, and grill the steaks for 3 to 4 minutes per side for medium-rare (130°F); cook for less or more time depending on your desired degree of doneness. A couple of minutes before the steaks are done, pour the reserved marinade over them and cook for 2 minutes to allow the shallots and garlic to flavor

231

the meat. Transfer the steaks to a cutting board and let rest while you grill the mushrooms.

Carefully arrange the mushrooms on the grill and cook, turning them occasionally, until tender, about 5 minutes total. Transfer the mushrooms to a platter, spreading them in an even layer.

Thinly slice the steaks on the bias and arrange the slices on the mushrooms. Drizzle with the remaining 2 tablespoons olive oil and serve.

Nutritional analysis per serving: Calories: 868, Fat: 37 g, Saturated Fat: 8 g, Cholesterol: 104 mg, Fiber: 68 g, Protein: 46 g, Carbohydrates: 109 g, Sodium: 395 mg

POT ROAST

Serves: 4

Prep time: 10 minutes

Cook time: 3 to 4 hours (unattended)

Fork-tender pot roast and vegetables moistened with an herb-infused sauce is comfort food at its finest. Serve this dish with Cauliflower "Rice" with Scallions (page 156) or mashed sweet potatoes.

- 1 (2-pound) beef bottom round roast
- 1 large yellow onion, roughly chopped
- 4 large carrots, scrubbed and cut into big chunks
- 4 cups cremini mushrooms, quartered
- 3 garlic cloves, minced
- 2 cups tomato puree
- 2 cups beef stock or filtered water
- 1 large bay leaf
- 2 sprigs thyme
- 1 teaspoon sea salt
- ½ teaspoon freshly ground black pepper

Preheat the oven to 325°F.

Place the beef in a large Dutch oven, then add the remaining ingredients. Set the pot over high heat and bring the liquid to a boil. Cover, place the pot in the oven, and cook, basting the roast with the cooking liquid every 20 to 30 minutes until the beef is fork-tender, 3 to 4 hours.

Remove the pot from the oven and transfer the roast to a cutting board. Allow to rest for a few minutes, then cut the roast against the grain into ¼-inch slices. Serve the pot roast and the vegetables moistened with the cooking liquid.

Nutritional analysis per serving: *Calories: 486, Fat: 9 g, Saturated Fat: 2 g, Cholesterol: 128 mg, Fiber: 6 g, Protein: 63 g, Carbohydrates: 42 g, Sodium: 811 mg*

Gingery Beef and Vegetable Stew with Coconut Milk

Serves: 4

Prep time:
20 minutes

Cook time:
2½ hours
(mostly
unattended)

In the winter, this stew is a staple for my family. It's easy to make, and so many of its ingredients are deeply nourishing. The ginger and coconut milk lend the dish an exotic aroma and flavor—they make this dish a nice change from the usual beef stew.

- 2 tablespoons Ghee (page 279)
- 2 large yellow onions, roughly chopped
- 3 garlic cloves, minced
- 1 (2-inch) piece ginger, peeled and minced
- 1 pound beef stew meat
- 2 large carrots, scrubbed and sliced into ¼-inch rounds
- 1 cup Coconut Milk (page 55)
- 1½ cups tomato puree
- 1 pound turnips, celery root, or rutabaga, peeled and cut into 1-inch chunks
- 1 bunch kale (any kind), stemmed and roughly chopped
- ¾ teaspoon sea salt

In a Dutch oven, warm the ghee over medium-high heat until shimmering. Add the onions and cook until softened and lightly browned, 3 to 4 minutes. Stir in the garlic and ginger, add the beef, and cook until the beef begins to brown, 2 to 3 minutes. Add the carrots, coconut milk, tomato puree, and 6 cups filtered water. Bring to a boil, then cover the pot, reduce the heat to medium-low, and simmer, stirring occasionally until the beef is tender, about 1½ hours.

Add the turnips, stir to combine, and continue to simmer until the turnips are tender, about 25 minutes. Stir in the kale and salt and cook until the kale is wilted and tender, about 5 minutes.

Spoon the stew into bowls and serve.

Nutritional analysis per serving: *Calories: 479, Fat: 26 g, Saturated Fat: 15 g, Cholesterol: 75 mg, Fiber: 6 g, Protein: 28 g, Carbohydrates: 34 g, Sodium: 685 mg*

BALSAMIC BEEF STEW

Serves: 4

Prep time:
5 minutes

Cook time:
2 hours

The combination of healthy fats, protein, vegetables, and herbs makes this recipe an all-around healthy hit. The addition of balsamic vinegar adds a sweet and sour flavor that beautifully blends into the stew. You can enjoy this recipe year-round, although winter is my favorite time to make this hearty stew.

- 2 tablespoons Ghee (page 279)
- 1 large yellow onion, roughly chopped
- 4 garlic cloves, minced
- 2 tablespoons tomato paste
- 1 cup dry red wine
- ¼ cup balsamic vinegar
- 1½ pounds beef stew meat
- 4 cups Dr. Hyman's Veggie-Bone Broth (page 128)
- 2 bay leaves
- 1 teaspoon dried thyme
- 2 carrots, scrubbed and cut into large chunks
- 3 celery ribs, diced
- 1 teaspoon sea salt

In a Dutch oven, warm the ghee over medium heat until melted. Add the onion and cook, stirring occasionally, until softened and translucent, about 5 minutes. Stir in the garlic and cook until fragrant, about 1 minute. Add the tomato paste and cook, stirring frequently to prevent it from burning, until the tomato paste darkens, about 2 minutes. Pour in the wine and balsamic vinegar and simmer until reduced by about half. Add the beef, bone broth, bay leaves, and thyme and stir to combine. Bring to a simmer, then cover partially and cook until the beef is tender, about 1½ hours.

Add the carrots and celery, stir to combine, and continue to cook until the carrots are tender, about 30 minutes. Remove and discard the bay leaves.

Stir in the salt. Spoon the stew into bowls and serve.

Nutritional analysis per serving: *Calories: 493, Fat: 27 g, Saturated Fat: 12 g, Cholesterol: 128 mg, Fiber: 2 g, Protein: 40 g, Carbohydrates: 15 g, Sodium: 618 mg*

ASIAN-SPICED BRAISED BEEF WITH BABY BOK CHOY

Serves: 5

Prep time:
20 minutes

Cook time:
3 hours

Tough cuts of meat, such as the top round used here, do best with slow cooking, which helps to break down the muscle fibers and create a tender, yielding texture. I've paired this Asian-inspired braised beef with baby bok choy, a vegetable with powerful antioxidants and anti-inflammatory properties.

- 1 tablespoon Ghee (page 279)
- 1 small yellow onion, minced
- 1 (2-inch) piece ginger, peeled and minced
- 1 (3-pound) beef top round
- 2 teaspoons ground cloves
- 1½ teaspoons ground cumin
- 1½ teaspoons ground fennel seeds
- 5 whole star anise
- 4 bay leaves
- 3 cinnamon sticks
- 2 cups chicken stock
- ¼ cup low-sodium, wheat-free tamari
- ¼ cup mirin
- 4 heads baby bok choy, halved lengthwise and cored
- 2 tablespoons toasted sesame seeds

Preheat the oven to 325°F.

In a Dutch oven, warm the ghee over medium-high heat until melted. Add the onion and cook, stirring occasionally, until softened and translucent, 3 to 4 minutes. Stir in the ginger and cook until fragrant, about 1 minute. Add the beef, cloves, cumin, fennel seeds, star anise, bay leaves, cinnamon sticks, chicken stock, tamari, and mirin. Bring to a boil, cover the pot, and place it in the oven. Cook, basting the beef every 20 to 30 minutes with the cooking liquid, until the meat is fork-tender and easily breaks apart, about 2½ hours.

Transfer the beef to a cutting board; reserve the cooking liquid in the pot. Using two forks, pull the meat into large shreds.

Fill a large saucepan with about 1 inch of water and place a steamer basket in the pan. Bring the water to a boil over high heat. Add the bok choy halves to the steamer basket and cook, covered, until tender, about 3 minutes.

Arrange the bok choy on a platter and top with the shredded beef. Pour the reserved cooking liquid through a fine-mesh sieve set over a bowl, then pour the liquid over the beef and bok choy. Sprinkle with the sesame seeds and serve.

Nutritional analysis per serving: Calories: 730, Fat: 26 g, Saturated Fat: 10 g, Cholesterol: 197 mg, Fiber: 6 g, Protein: 84 g, Carbohydrates: 29 g, Sodium: 554 mg

SLOW-COOKER BEEF STEW WITH CABBAGE, CARROTS, AND MUSHROOMS

Serves: 4

Prep time: 20 minutes

Cook time: 8 to 10 hours (unattended)

The slow cooker is the perfect tool for those of us who are challenged by a schedule that makes it difficult to prepare healthful home-cooked dinners on weeknights. With this recipe, all you need to do is put the ingredients in the slow cooker in the morning, and when you return in the evening, dinner will be ready.

- 1 large yellow onion, roughly chopped
- 2 large carrots, scrubbed and cut into ¼-inch rounds
- 3 celery ribs, cut into ½-inch pieces
- 3 cups button mushrooms, quartered
- 1 (2-pound) head green cabbage, cut into 8 wedges and cored
- 4 garlic cloves, thinly sliced
- 2 bay leaves
- 1 (2- by 6-inch) strip dried kelp, snipped into small pieces
- 1 pound beef stew meat
- 1 (15-ounce) can diced fire-roasted tomatoes
- 4 cups chicken stock
- ½ teaspoon freshly ground black pepper
- ½ bunch parsley, stemmed and roughly chopped
- 8 tablespoons unsalted, grass-fed butter, at room temperature

In a large slow cooker, combine the onion, carrots, celery, mushrooms, cabbage, garlic, bay leaves, kelp, beef, tomatoes with their juice, chicken stock, and pepper. Set the temperature to low and cook until the beef is fork-tender, 8 to 10 hours.

Remove and discard the bay leaves. Stir the parsley into the stew. Spoon the stew into 4 bowls, evenly dividing the beef and vegetables. Top each portion with 2 tablespoons of the butter and serve.

Nutritional analysis per serving: *Calories: 576, Fat: 39 g, Saturated Fat: 16 g, Cholesterol: 136 mg, Fiber: 8 g, Protein: 29 g, Carbohydrates: 31 g, Sodium: 640 mg*

BRAISED SHORT RIBS WITH FENNEL SEED AND CIDER VINEGAR

Serves: 4

Prep time:
5 minutes

Cook time:
2¾ hours
(mostly
unattended)

Short ribs are the perfect example of how a tough cut of meat can be transformed by cooking slow and low. A few hours in the oven and the ribs become fork-tender and succulent, and they absorb the flavors of the ingredients cooked with them. Bone broth as a braising liquid adds healing properties and lots of nutritional value to this rich and satisfying dish.

- 4 large bone-in beef short ribs
- 3 garlic cloves, minced
- 1 cup tomato puree
- 2 cups Dr. Hyman's Veggie-Bone Broth (page 128)
- 1 tablespoon Dijon mustard
- 2 teaspoons ground fennel seeds
- ¼ cup apple cider vinegar
- ¾ teaspoon sea salt

Preheat the oven to 325°F.

Combine all the ingredients in a Dutch oven and bring to a boil over medium-high heat. Cover the pot, place it in the oven, and cook until the meat is fork-tender, about 2½ hours.

Carefully transfer the short ribs to 4 shallow serving bowls. Using a spoon, skim off and discard as much fat as you can from the surface of the cooking liquid. Pour the cooking liquid into a blender and blend on high speed until smooth, about 45 seconds. Pour the sauce over the short ribs, dividing it evenly, and serve. Pairs nicely with cauliflower or sweet potato mash and a side of greens.

Nutritional analysis per serving: *Calories: 442, Fat: 37 g, Saturated Fat: 16 g, Cholesterol: 84 mg, Fiber: 2 g, Protein: 18 g, Carbohydrates: 7 g, Sodium: 608 mg*

Buffalo Burgers with Kelp Powder

Serves: 4

Prep time:
5 minutes

Cook time:
10 minutes

Kelp, a natural detoxifier, is a wild ocean plant loaded with minerals. It has an earthy, savory flavor that works perfectly with the seasonings in these burgers. Ground buffalo is readily available these days, but if you can't find it, use grass-fed beef or lamb instead.

- 1 pound ground buffalo
- 1 tablespoon onion powder
- 2 teaspoons paprika
- 2 teaspoons dried kelp powder
- 1½ teaspoons dried thyme
- 1 teaspoon dried oregano
- 1 teaspoon garlic powder
- 1 teaspoon sea salt
- olive oil, for greasing the grill grate (if using a charcoal or gas grill)

In a bowl, combine all the ingredients except the oil and mix until thoroughly combined. Divide the mixture into 4 portions and shape each into a 3-inch patty.

Heat a large, well-seasoned stove-top grill pan over medium-high heat. Alternatively, build a medium-hot fire in a charcoal grill or preheat a gas grill to medium-high; when the grill is hot, scrape the grate clean and lightly grease it with olive oil. Grill the burgers for 3 to 4 minutes per side for medium-rare (130°F); cook for less or more time depending on your desired degree of doneness. Serve.

Nutritional analysis per serving: Calories: 269, Fat: 12 g, Saturated Fat: 4 g, Cholesterol: 50 mg, Fiber: 11 g, Protein: 23 g, Carbohydrates: 20 g, Sodium: 909 mg

SHEPHERD'S PIE

Serves: 6

Prep time: 30 minutes

Cook time: 45 minutes

In this recipe, mashed carrots and sweet potatoes stand in for the basic mashed potatoes that top a traditional shepherd's pie, giving this comfort-food classic a nutritional boost. This dish freezes nicely, so make it ahead and keep it on hand for those times when you're too busy to cook.

- 1 pound carrots, scrubbed and cut into 1-inch pieces
- 1 pound sweet potatoes, peeled and cut into 1-inch chunks
- 1 tablespoon unsalted, grass-fed butter
- ½ teaspoon sea salt
- 1 tablespoon Ghee (page 279)
- 2 pounds ground lamb
- ½ large yellow onion, minced
- 2 teaspoons garlic powder
- 1 cup Dr. Hyman's Veggie-Bone Broth (page 128) or filtered water
- 2 tablespoons arrowroot
- 1 teaspoon minced fresh rosemary

In a medium saucepan, combine the carrots and sweet potatoes and pour in 2 cups filtered water. Cover, bring to a boil over medium-high heat, and cook until the vegetables are tender, about 8 minutes. Drain the vegetables in a colander and return them to the pan. Using a potato masher, mash the vegetables until smooth. Stir in the butter and salt. Cover to keep warm and set aside.

While the carrots and sweet potatoes cook, in a large skillet, warm the ghee over medium-high heat until melted. Add the lamb and cook, stirring occasionally, until it begins to brown, about 2 minutes. Add the onion and continue to cook, stirring occasionally, until the onion begins to soften, 3 to 4 minutes. Stir in the garlic powder, pour in the bone broth, and bring to a boil. Reduce the heat to medium and simmer until the lamb is cooked through, about 5 minutes. In a small bowl, mix the arrowroot with 2 tablespoons filtered water. Stir the arrowroot mixture into the lamb mixture, increase the heat to medium-high, and bring to a boil, stirring constantly, to thicken the liquid. Stir in the rosemary and remove from the heat.

Preheat the broiler.

Pour the lamb mixture into a 9- by 13-inch broiler-safe baking dish, then jiggle the dish to distribute the mixture in an even layer. Using a spatula, spread the carrot–sweet potato mash in an even layer over the lamb. Broil the shepherd's pie until the top is golden brown, 2 to 3 minutes.

Cut the pie into squares and serve.

Nutritional analysis per serving: *Calories: 591, Fat: 41 g, Saturated Fat: 18 g, Cholesterol: 118 mg, Fiber: 5 g, Protein: 27 g, Carbohydrates: 28 g, Sodium: 381 mg*

GRILLED LAMB CHOPS WITH FRESH MINT AND BABA GHANOUSH

Serves: 4

Prep time: 15 minutes

Cook time: 1 hour

Baba ghanoush is a Middle Eastern eggplant puree flavored with tahini, lemon, and olive oil. This version includes parsley, tomato, and capers for added color and flavor. Though baba ghanoush is often served as a dip, here it's a wonderful side dish to simple grilled lamb chops.

- 2 large globe eggplants
- 3 garlic cloves
- ½ bunch parsley, stemmed
- ¼ cup tahini, plus more if needed
- 2 tablespoons fresh lemon juice, plus more if needed
- 1 teaspoon sea salt
- 1 small tomato, roughly chopped
- 2 teaspoons drained capers, minced
- 8 bone-in lamb loin chops
- 4 tablespoons extra-virgin olive oil, plus more for greasing the grill grate
- ½ teaspoon freshly ground black pepper
- ¼ cup fresh mint leaves, thinly sliced

Preheat the oven to 375°F.

To make the baba ghanoush, poke the eggplants all over with a fork. Place the eggplants on a baking sheet and bake until softened and collapsed, 20 to 30 minutes. Allow the eggplants to cool completely.

Set a fine-mesh sieve over a bowl. Cut open the eggplants and use a spoon to scoop the flesh from the skins into the sieve; discard the skins. Let drain for 5 minutes, then transfer the eggplant to a food processor. Add the garlic, parsley, tahini, lemon juice, and ½ teaspoon of the salt. Pulse a few times to combine, then process until the mixture is smooth and creamy, about 1 minute. Taste and add more tahini or lemon juice to suit your preference. Transfer the puree to a bowl, then fold in the tomato and capers. Cover and refrigerate until ready to serve.

Build a medium-hot fire in a charcoal grill or preheat a gas grill to medium-high.

Drizzle the lamb chops with 2 tablespoons of the olive oil and season with the remaining salt and the pepper. Scrape the grill grate clean and lightly grease it with olive oil. Grill the chops for about 3 minutes per side for medium-rare (130°F); cook for less or more time depending on your desired degree of doneness.

Place 2 lamb chops on each of 4 plates and spoon baba ghanoush alongside the chops. Sprinkle each serving with 1 tablespoon of the mint leaves, drizzle with 1½ teaspoons of the remaining olive oil, and serve.

Nutritional analysis per serving: Calories: 418, Fat: 30 g, Saturated Fat: 7 g, Cholesterol: 0 mg, Fiber: 9 g, Protein: 20 g, Carbohydrates: 21 g, Sodium: 688 mg

LAMB MEATBALLS WITH TOMATO-CUCUMBER SALAD AND CASHEW "YOGURT"

Serves: 4

Prep time: 20 minutes, plus standing and chilling time

Cook time: 15 minutes

With classic Middle Eastern flavors, these lamb meatballs make a great lunch or dinner. Make the cashew "yogurt" at least one day before you plan to serve the dish because it must stand at room temperature for several hours to allow the cashew to ferment like real yogurt. After it sits at room temperature, you can chill the "yogurt" in the refrigerator.

- ½ cup raw cashews
- 1 tablespoon fresh lemon juice
- 2 tablespoons extra-virgin olive oil
- 1 pound ground lamb
- ½ cup loosely packed fresh parsley leaves, roughly chopped
- ¼ cup loosely packed fresh mint leaves, roughly chopped
- 2 large sprigs oregano, leaves only, finely chopped
- 3 garlic cloves, minced
- ¼ teaspoon crushed red pepper flakes
- 1 tablespoon chia seeds, ground in a spice grinder
- 1 pint cherry tomatoes, cut in half
- 1 cucumber, peeled and sliced into ¼-inch rounds
- 2 scallions, thinly sliced
- 1 tablespoon apple cider vinegar
- sprinkle of fresh dill, for garnish (optional)

To make the cashew "yogurt," combine the cashews, lemon juice, and 6 tablespoons filtered water in a blender and blend on high speed until smooth and creamy, about 1 minute; add more water as needed to achieve a yogurt–like consistency. Pour the mixture into a glass container, cover, and let stand at room temperature for 8 to 12 hours, then refrigerate until cold, at least 1 hour or up to 3 days.

Preheat the oven to 350°F. Drizzle a 9- by 13-inch baking dish with 1 tablespoon of the olive oil.

To make the meatballs, in a medium bowl, combine the lamb, parsley, mint, oregano, garlic, red pepper flakes, and chia seeds. Mix well. Form the mixture into 12 evenly sized balls and place them in the prepared baking dish. Bake until firm, 10 to 12 minutes.

To make the salad, in a large bowl, combine the tomatoes, cucumber, and scallions. Drizzle with the vinegar and the remaining 1 tablespoon olive oil, and toss well.

Divide the salad among 4 plates. Place 3 meatballs alongside the salad on each plate, drizzle generously with cashew "yogurt," sprinkle on some fresh dill, if using, and serve.

Nutritional analysis per serving: *Calories: 779, Fat: 68 g, Saturated Fat: 18 g, Cholesterol: 83 mg, Fiber: 4 g, Protein: 27 g, Carbohydrates: 20 g, Sodium: 89 mg*

CARIBBEAN LAMB STEW

Serves: 4

Prep time:
10 minutes

Cook time:
2 hours

When shopping, look for grass-fed lamb, one of the most nutritious animal proteins available because of the omega-3s and vitamin B$_{12}$ it contains. The ginger, curry, coconut, and especially the allspice give this stew a Caribbean flavor profile. Serve Cauliflower "Rice" with Scallions (page 156) on the side.

- 1 tablespoon coconut oil
- 1 pound lamb stew meat
- 1 large yellow onion, chopped
- 1 (1-inch) piece ginger, peeled and minced
- 1 tablespoon curry powder
- ½ teaspoon ground allspice
- 2 cups tomato puree
- 1 (13.5-ounce) can full-fat coconut milk
- 1 cup Dr. Hyman's Veggie-Bone Broth (page 128)
- ½ teaspoon sea salt
- sprinkle of parsley, for garnish (optional)

In a large saucepan, warm the coconut oil over medium-high heat until shimmering. Add the lamb and cook, stirring occasionally, until lightly browned on all sides, 3 to 4 minutes. Add the onion and cook, stirring occasionally, until the onion begins to soften, about 2 minutes. Stir in the ginger, curry, and allspice, then pour in the tomato puree, coconut milk, and bone broth. Bring to a boil, then reduce the heat to medium, partially cover, and simmer, stirring occasionally, until the lamb is fork-tender, about 2 hours. Stir in the salt.

Divide the stew among 4 serving bowls, sprinkle with the parsley, if using, and serve.

Nutritional analysis per serving: Calories: 657, Fat: 36 g, Saturated Fat: 23 g, Cholesterol: 151 mg, Fiber: 9 g, Protein: 52 g, Carbohydrates: 38 g, Sodium: 401 mg

Braised Lamb Shanks with Moroccan Flavors

Serves: 4

Prep time:
10 minutes

Cook time:
4 hours (mostly
unattended)

Bring out those spices and put them to good use in this lamb dish inspired by Moroccan flavors. Not only do spices add flavor and fragrance to your meals; they also contain phytochemicals that can strengthen your immune system. So why not add a little spice to your life?

- 2 tablespoons Ghee (page 279)
- 1 large yellow onion, finely chopped
- 3 large garlic cloves, minced
- 2 teaspoons paprika
- 1½ teaspoons ground cumin
- 1 teaspoon ground coriander
- ⅛ teaspoon saffron threads
- 4 (8-ounce) lamb shanks
- 1 preserved lemon, thinly sliced
- 4 large carrots, scrubbed and quartered crosswise
- ½ bunch cilantro, stemmed and roughly chopped
- ½ teaspoon sea salt
- ½ teaspoon freshly ground black pepper

In a Dutch oven, warm the ghee over medium heat until shimmering. Add the onion and cook, stirring occasionally, until softened and translucent, about 5 minutes. Stir in the garlic and cook until fragrant, about 1 minute, then stir in the paprika, cumin, coriander, and saffron and cook until the spices are fragrant, about 2 minutes. Place the lamb shanks in a single layer on top of the onion mixture. Pour in enough filtered water to submerge the shanks about halfway. Bring to a boil, then reduce the heat to low, partially cover, and simmer, basting and flipping the shanks about every 30 minutes, until the lamb is tender, about 3 hours.

Stir in the preserved lemon slices and carrots. Cover the pot and cook, basting the shanks about every 15 minutes, until the carrots are tender, about 30 minutes. Stir in the cilantro, salt, and pepper.

Arrange one shank in each of 4 shallow bowls, place the carrots and lemons alongside, and spoon sauce over each portion. Serve.

Nutritional analysis per serving: *Calories: 576, Fat: 27 g, Saturated Fat: 11 g, Cholesterol: 202 mg, Fiber: 1 g, Protein: 66 g, Carbohydrates: 13 g, Sodium: 695 mg*

14

Breads and Desserts

SPICED SWEET POTATO QUICK BREAD

Easy to make and naturally sweet from the sweet potatoes, this quick bread is perfect whenever you need a bread fix. It's especially good slathered with softened ghee or butter.

- 2 tablespoons coconut oil
- 2 large sweet potatoes, peeled and thinly sliced
- ½ cup coconut flour
- 1 tablespoon ground cinnamon
- 1 teaspoon ground nutmeg
- ½ teaspoon ground mace
- 1 teaspoon baking soda
- 1 teaspoon baking powder
- ⅛ teaspoon sea salt
- 4 large eggs
- ½ cup almond butter
- 4 tablespoons unsalted, grass-fed butter, melted
- 1 teaspoon organic almond extract

Makes: 1
(9- by 5-inch)
loaf

Prep time:
10 minutes

Cook time:
1 hour

Preheat the oven to 350°F. Grease a 9- by 5-inch loaf pan with the coconut oil. Cut a piece of parchment paper to fit in the bottom of the pan and lay the parchment in the pan.

Place the sweet potato slices in a medium saucepan and cover with about 1 inch filtered water. Bring to a boil over high heat and cook until tender, about 5 minutes. Drain the potatoes in a colander, then return the slices to the saucepan. Using a potato masher, mash the potatoes until smooth and allow to cool to room temperature.

In a bowl, combine the coconut flour, cinnamon, nutmeg, mace, baking soda, baking powder, and salt.

In a large bowl, whisk the eggs until combined. Add the mashed sweet potatoes and the almond butter, melted butter, and almond extract and whisk gently until well combined. Add the coconut flour mixture and mix with a rubber spatula until evenly moistened. Pour the batter into the prepared loaf pan and bake until a toothpick inserted into the center comes out clean, 50 to 60 minutes.

Invert the bread out of the pan onto a wire rack and allow to cool completely. Cut the loaf into 1-inch slices and serve. Store tightly wrapped in plastic wrap at room temperature for up to 4 days.

Nutritional analysis per serving (1 slice): Calories: 405, Fat: 19 g, Saturated Fat: 7 g, Cholesterol: 95 mg, Fiber: 43 g, Protein: 9 g, Carbohydrates: 70 g, Sodium: 323 mg

INJERA (ETHIOPIAN FLATBREAD)

PEGAN DIET

Makes: about 8 (6-inch) injeras

Prep time: 5 minutes, plus 1 to 2 days for fermentation

Cook time: 10 minutes

Injera is a traditional food of Ethiopia. This soft, spongy bread is made with gluten-free teff flour, and fermentation gives it a tangy flavor. Serve the rounds of bread with any meal, use them as a base for your morning eggs, or simply spread them with butter and enjoy.

- 3 cups teff flour
- 2 teaspoons sea salt
- 4 tablespoons Ghee (page 279) or extra-virgin olive oil, for cooking

In a large bowl, combine the teff flour and salt, pour in 4 cups filtered water, and whisk to combine. The mixture should resemble loose pancake batter. Cover the bowl with a clean kitchen towel and allow to stand at room temperature until small bubbles form in the batter, 1 to 2 days.

In a well-seasoned 8-inch cast-iron skillet, warm 1½ teaspoons ghee over medium heat until shimmering. Add about ¼ cup of the batter to the center of the pan, use a spatula to spread it out into a 6-inch round, and cook until completely dry on the surface, 4 to 5 minutes. Transfer the injera to a large plate. Cook the remaining batter in the same way, using additional ghee and stacking the injera on the plate.

Serve the injera at room temperature. Refrigerate leftovers in a large ziplock bag with paper towels between layers for up to 4 days.

Nutritional analysis per serving (1 round bread): *Calories: 237, Fat: 9 g, Saturated Fat: 5 g, Cholesterol: 15 mg, Fiber: 6 g, Protein: 6 g, Carbohydrates: 33 g, Sodium: 568 mg*

Lemon-Cashew "Curd" with Fresh Blueberries

Serves: 4

Prep time:
20 minutes,
plus soaking
and chilling
time

PEGAN DIET

When wild blueberries ripen in the late summer, I always look forward to picking—and eating!—the tiny fruits. Blueberries are loaded with antioxidants and deliver a pleasant balance of sweet and tart flavors. This lemony, blueberry-garnished cashew "curd" comes together easily in a blender and is a light, refreshing dessert.

- 2 cups raw cashews
- ½ cup unsweetened cashew milk or filtered water
- ¼ cup fresh lemon juice
- grated zest of 2 lemons
- ½ teaspoon vanilla powder
- 1 tablespoon maple syrup
- 1 cup blueberries
- ¼ cup bee pollen

Put the cashews in a medium bowl and cover with 4 cups filtered water. Let soak at room temperature for 30 minutes.

Drain the cashews and rinse well. In a blender, combine the cashews, cashew milk, lemon juice and zest, vanilla powder, and maple syrup. Blend on high speed until the mixture is very smooth and creamy, about 1 minute.

Divide the "curd" among 4 wineglasses or dessert bowls. Cover and refrigerate until chilled, at least 2 hours or up to 8 hours.

Top each portion of chilled "curd" with ¼ cup of the blueberries, sprinkle with 1 tablespoon of the bee pollen, and serve.

Nutritional analysis per serving: Calories: 431, Fat: 30 g, Saturated Fat: 6 g, Cholesterol: 0 mg, Fiber: 6 g, Protein: 15 g, Carbohydrates: 35 g, Sodium: 3 mg, Sugars: 9 g

PANNA COTTA WITH BLUEBERRIES AND PECANS

Serves: 4

Prep time:
30 minutes,
plus cooling
time

Cook time:
10 minutes

Panna cotta is a traditional Italian dessert with a custard-like texture. Its name translates to "cooked cream," but this version uses coconut milk. Blueberries and pecans hide at the bottom of each ramekin for a delicious surprise.

- ¾ cup fresh or thawed frozen blueberries
- ¼ cup toasted pecans, roughly chopped
- 2 (13.5-ounce) cans full-fat coconut milk
- 2 tablespoons unflavored powdered gelatin
- 1 teaspoon ground cinnamon
- ½ teaspoon vanilla powder

If using thawed frozen blueberries, drain them in a fine-mesh sieve to remove excess moisture.

In a small bowl, stir together the blueberries and pecans, then divide the mixture evenly among 4 (1-cup) ramekins.

Pour the coconut milk into a medium saucepan, then sprinkle the gelatin over the top. Allow to stand until the gelatin swells, about 5 minutes. Set the pan over low heat and warm the mixture, whisking constantly, just until the gelatin dissolves. Remove from the heat and stir in the cinnamon and vanilla powder. Pour the mixture into the ramekins, dividing it evenly, cover, and refrigerate until chilled and set, at least 4 hours or up to 8 hours.

Serve the chilled panna cotta in the ramekins.

Nutritional analysis per serving: *Calories: 291, Fat: 26 g, Saturated Fat: 18 g, Cholesterol: 0 mg, Fiber: 2 g, Protein: 6 g, Carbohydrates: 10 g, Sodium: 43 mg*

Chocolate-Avocado Pudding with Cinnamon

Serves: 4

Prep time: 30 minutes, plus chilling time

PEGAN DIET

People often associate healthful eating with a lack of flavor. This dessert will convince skeptics that that doesn't have to be the case! Rich and creamy avocado is transformed into a simple no-cook pudding that will satisfy any chocolate lover's craving.

- 1 cup unsweetened Nut Milk (page 54)
- 4 Medjool dates, pitted
- 2 avocados, pitted and peeled
- ⅓ cup cacao powder
- 1 teaspoon pure vanilla extract
- 1 teaspoon ground cinnamon
- ⅛ teaspoon sea salt
- 1 cup raspberries

In a small saucepan, warm the nut milk over low heat until just shy of simmering. Add the dates, remove the pan from the heat, and allow to cool to room temperature. (You can speed up the cooling process by transferring the nut milk and dates to a bowl and refrigerating.)

Scoop the softened dates out of the nut milk and place them in a food processor; reserve the milk. Pulse until the dates are broken up, about 6 pulses. Scrape down the sides of the bowl, add the avocados, and pulse until the avocados are mostly smashed, 4 or 5 pulses, scraping down the bowl as needed. Add the cacao powder, vanilla, cinnamon, salt, and reserved nut milk and process until the mixture is smooth and creamy.

Divide the pudding among 4 (⅓-cup) ramekins or dessert bowls. Cover and refrigerate until chilled, at least 1 hour or up to 8 hours.

Top the puddings with the raspberries, dividing them evenly, and serve.

Nutritional analysis per serving: *Calories: 395, Fat: 13 g, Saturated Fat: 2 g, Cholesterol: 0 mg, Fiber: 40 g, Protein: 6 g, Carbohydrates: 82 g, Sodium: 129 mg, Sugars: 20 g*

CHOCOLATE-PISTACHIO FUDGE

PEGAN DIET

Makes: 12
(2-inch) pieces

Prep time:
15 minutes, plus
chilling time

Chocolate makes me happy: It tastes amazing *and* it's filled with antioxidants. This recipe combines chocolate, coconut milk, pistachios, and cardamom to create an easy-to-make fudge with exotic flavors that you don't have to feel guilty about eating.

- 12 ounces bittersweet chocolate, 70% or higher, finely chopped
- 1 teaspoon vanilla powder
- ½ teaspoon ground cardamom
- ¼ teaspoon sea salt
- 1 tablespoon Ghee (page 279)
- 1 cup full-fat coconut milk
- 2 tablespoons maple sugar
- ¼ cup shelled raw pistachios, roughly chopped
- cacao powder, for dusting

Line a baking sheet with parchment paper.

In a large heatproof bowl, combine the chopped chocolate, vanilla, cardamom, and salt.

In a small saucepan, combine the ghee, coconut milk, and maple sugar and warm over medium-low heat, stirring to dissolve the sugar, until just shy of simmering, then immediately pour the mixture over the chocolate. Stir until the chocolate is completely melted and the mixture is smooth and very thick. Gently stir in the pistachios.

Transfer the mixture to the prepared baking sheet and use a spatula to form it as best as you can into a 6- by 8-inch slab about ½ inch thick. Refrigerate until the fudge is firm, at least 12 hours, or freeze for about 4 hours.

Cut the chilled slab into 12 (2-inch) squares, dust with cacao powder, and serve. Store in an airtight container in the refrigerator for up to 7 days.

Nutritional analysis per serving (1 piece): *Calories: 115, Fat: 7 g, Saturated Fat: 4 g, Cholesterol: 508 mg, Fiber: 0 g, Protein: 14 g, Carbohydrates: 1 g, Sodium: 426 mg, Sugars: 6 g*

CHOCOLATE TRUFFLES

Makes:
20 truffles

Prep time:
20 minutes,
plus chilling
time

PEGAN DIET

Sweetened with dates, these little confections will satisfy when the craving strikes for something rich and chocolaty. If you'd like to change up the flavor a bit, dust the tops of the cacao-coated truffles with ground cinnamon or ground seeds—or even curry powder for a spicy kick!

- 7 to 9 Medjool dates, pitted
- 1 cup raw cashews
- 3 tablespoons cacao powder, plus ¼ cup for dusting
- 1 teaspoon alcohol-free, gluten-free pure vanilla extract
- 1 teaspoon ground nutmeg
- ⅛ teaspoon sea salt

In a food processor, combine 7 of the dates, the cashews, 3 tablespoons of the cacao powder, and the vanilla, nutmeg, and salt. Process until the mixture is finely ground and begins to stick together, 45 to 60 seconds. Pinch off a marble-size piece and squeeze it in your hand; it should be cohesive. If it isn't, return it to the food processor, add the remaining 2 dates, and process until well combined.

Transfer the mixture to a bowl. Using a small ice cream scoop or two spoons, portion the mixture into 20 evenly sized mounds and place on a small baking sheet. Use your hands to roll each mound, one at a time, into a firmly packed ball and place it back on the baking sheet.

Put the remaining cacao powder in a small bowl. Roll each truffle in the cacao powder until coated on all sides and return it to the baking sheet. Cover and refrigerate the truffles until firm, at least 1 hour or up to 1 week. Serve chilled.

Nutritional analysis per serving (1 truffle): Calories: 588, Fat: 58 g, Saturated Fat: 31 g, Cholesterol: 0 mg, Fiber: 3 g, Protein: 3 g, Carbohydrates: 12 g, Sodium: 60 mg, Sugars: 8 g

NO-BAKE WALNUT BROWNIES

PEGAN DIET

Everybody loves a good brownie, but most are full of refined sugar and wheat flour. I've created a simple, no-bake version made with walnuts, impressively nutritious nuts that contain generous amounts of essential vitamins and minerals.

- 4 cups raw walnuts
- 1 cup cacao nibs
- ¼ cup cacao powder
- 2 Medjool dates, pitted
- 2 tablespoons unsalted, grass-fed butter, room temperature
- 3 tablespoons melted cacao butter
- pinch of sea salt

Makes:
8 (2-inch)
brownies

Prep time:
15 minutes,
plus chilling
time

Line the bottom of a 9-inch square baking dish with parchment paper.

In a food processor, combine all the ingredients and process until the mixture is well combined and free of large chunks (it will be grainy), about 45 seconds.

Transfer the mixture to the prepared baking dish and, using your hands, press it into an even, firmly packed layer. Cover and refrigerate until firm, at least 2 hours or up to 4 days. The brownies can also be frozen for up to 3 months.

Cut the chilled brownies into 2-inch pieces and serve.

Nutritional analysis per serving (1 brownie): *Calories: 560, Fat: 48 g, Saturated Fat: 5 g, Cholesterol: 8 mg, Fiber: 4 g, Protein: 24 g, Carbohydrates: 18 g, Sodium: 28 mg, Sugars: 4 g*

Buckwheat and Apple Crepes with Cashew Cream

Serves: 4

Prep time:
5 minutes, plus
resting time for
the batter

Cook time:
15 minutes

PEGAN DIET

This hearty, comforting dessert is perfect for the fall, when apples are in season. Buckwheat flour has a delicious, nutty flavor that pairs perfectly with the maple sugar and cashew cream in this recipe. These crepes are best hot out of the pan, so serve them as they are ready.

- 2 cups buckwheat flour
- 2 tablespoons maple sugar
- 1 teaspoon ground cinnamon
- ½ teaspoon ground ginger
- grated zest of 1 lemon
- ¼ teaspoon sea salt
- 2 large eggs, beaten
- ½ cup unsweetened almond milk
- 4 tablespoons unsalted, grass-fed butter, melted and cooled, plus more for cooking
- ½ cup cashews
- ¼ teaspoon vanilla powder
- 2 large crisp, tart apples

To make the crepe batter, in a bowl, whisk together the buckwheat flour, maple sugar, cinnamon, ground ginger, lemon zest, and salt. Whisk in the eggs and almond milk, then fold in the melted butter. Cover and set aside at room temperature for up to 1 hour or refrigerate for up to 2 days.

To make the cashew cream, add the cashews to a blender along with the vanilla powder and ½ cup filtered water. Blend on high for about 45 seconds, until creamy and free of lumps, adding more water if needed, until the cream is quite thick but runny. Transfer the cream to a jar, cover, and store in the fridge until ready to serve.

When you're ready to cook and serve the crepes, peel, core, and slice the apples into thin wedges.

In an 8-inch skillet, warm 1 tablespoon butter over medium heat until melted. Pour ¼ cup of the batter into the center of the skillet and use a spatula to spread the batter into a 4-inch circle about ¼ inch thick. Carefully arrange one-fourth of the apple slices in a pinwheel shape on the batter and cook until the crepe is lightly browned on the bottom, about 2 minutes. Using a metal spatula, carefully flip the crepe and cook until done, 2 to 3 minutes, adding more butter as needed to prevent sticking. Flip the crepe onto a plate so that the apples are facing up, top with cashew cream, and serve.

Make 3 more crepes using the remaining batter and apple slices, topping each with cashew cream before serving.

Nutritional analysis per serving: *Calories: 503, Fat: 18 g, Saturated Fat: 9 g, Cholesterol: 123 mg, Fiber: 13 g, Protein: 14 g, Carbohydrates: 80 g, Sodium: 219 mg, Sugars: 17 g*

RASPBERRY-COCONUT ICE CREAM

Serves: 4

Prep time:
5 minutes

Ice cream made with frozen fruit and coconut cream is every bit as rich and delicious as dairy-based ice cream. Here I use raspberries, which are a fantastic source of vitamin C and fiber. You don't need an ice cream machine for this recipe, but for best results, use a high-speed blender that comes with a tamper so the berries puree thoroughly and the mixture is quick to turn smooth and creamy. The ice cream doesn't keep well, so be prepared to serve all of it immediately after blending.

- 2 (10-ounce) packages frozen raspberries
- ½ cup coconut cream
- 1 teaspoon alcohol-free, gluten-free pure vanilla extract
- ½ teaspoon ground cardamom
- 2 tablespoons dark maple syrup (optional, for Pegan Diet)
- 2 tablespoons bee pollen
- 2 tablespoons shredded unsweetened coconut
- 2 tablespoons cacao nibs

Combine the raspberries, coconut cream, vanilla, cardamom, and maple syrup, if using, in a blender and blend on high speed, using the tamper (if available) to push the berries down toward the blade, until the mixture is smooth, thick, and creamy, about 1 minute.

Using a spatula, scoop the ice cream into 4 bowls. Sprinkle each portion with 1½ teaspoons each of the bee pollen, coconut, and cacao nibs and serve.

Nutritional analysis per serving: *Calories: 173, Fat: 3 g, Saturated Fat: 2 g, Cholesterol: 0 mg, Fiber: 12 g, Protein: 4 g, Carbohydrates: 26 g, Sodium: 8 mg, Sugars: 8 g*

PEACH ICE CREAM

PEGAN DIET

Serves: 4

Prep time: 10 minutes

The combination of peaches and cream is a southern classic, but here, coconut cream stands in for the dairy. As with the Raspberry-Coconut Ice Cream (page 262), you don't need an ice cream machine to make this dessert, but a high-speed blender works best to quickly and efficiently blend the mixture to a smooth, creamy consistency.

- 4 cups frozen peach slices
- ½ cup coconut cream
- ¼ cup coconut oil, softened
- 1 teaspoon vanilla powder
- 1 teaspoon ground mace
- ¼ cup cacao nibs

Working in 2 batches, combine the peach slices, coconut cream, coconut oil, vanilla powder, and mace in a blender and blend on high speed, using the tamper (if available) to push the peaches down toward the blade, until the mixture is smooth, thick, and creamy, about 1 minute. Transfer the mixture to a bowl and place the bowl in the freezer. Repeat with the remaining peaches, coconut cream, coconut oil, vanilla, and mace, mixing this second batch into the first batch in the freezer.

Scoop the ice cream into 4 bowls. Sprinkle each portion with 1 tablespoon of the cacao nibs and serve.

Nutritional analysis per serving: *Calories: 256, Fat: 25 g, Saturated Fat: 2 g, Cholesterol: 0 mg, Fiber: 4 g, Protein: 3 g, Carbohydrates: 19 g, Sodium: 5 mg*

15

Sauces, Condiments, and Seasonings

HOMEMADE MAYONNAISE

Makes: 1 cup

Prep time:
25 minutes

Once you taste homemade mayonnaise, you'll want to toss out the store-bought stuff in your refrigerator. If you choose to make the mayo by hand, you'll get a great arm workout because of all the vigorous whisking involved. Or you can make it in a blender with ease.

- 2 large egg yolks
- 1 tablespoon fresh lemon juice, plus more as needed
- 1 tablespoon white wine vinegar or champagne vinegar
- ¼ teaspoon Dijon mustard
- 1 teaspoon sea salt
- freshly ground white pepper
- 1 cup avocado oil or extra-virgin olive oil

To make the mayonnaise by hand, in a medium bowl, combine the egg yolks, lemon juice, vinegar, mustard, salt, and a pinch of white pepper. Stabilize the bowl by nestling the base in a bunched-up damp kitchen towel. Whisk the ingredients until well combined. While whisking continuously and vigorously, add the oil only a few drops at a time. Once the mixture starts to thicken, add the remaining oil in a very slow, thin stream while continuing to whisk. If you add too much oil too quickly, the mixture will not thicken, so it's better to go slow. You can stop for a moment to rest your arm or switch hands, if needed. After all the oil has been added, taste the mayonnaise and adjust the seasoning with pepper and/or lemon juice.

To make the mayonnaise in a blender, in a small bowl whisk together the egg yolks, lemon juice, vinegar, mustard, salt, and a pinch of white pepper until well combined. Transfer the mixture to a blender and blend on low speed for a few seconds. With the machine running, add the oil only a few drops at a time. Once the mixture starts to thicken, add the remaining oil in a very slow, thin stream. After all the oil has been added, taste the mayonnaise and adjust the seasoning with pepper and/or lemon juice.

Transfer the mayonnaise to a nonreactive container. Use right away or cover tightly and refrigerate for up to 4 days. If the mayonnaise gets too thick, whisk in up to 2 teaspoons cold filtered water to thin it.

Nutritional analysis per serving (1 tablespoon): *Calories: 100, Fat: 11 g, Saturated Fat: 2 g, Cholesterol: 25 mg, Fiber: 0 g, Protein: 0 g, Carbohydrates: 0 g, Sodium: 10 mg*

CHIPOTLE MAYONNAISE

You don't have to use the same old spreads and dips on this plan. Switch it up with this smoky chipotle mayonnaise that you'll want to spread on everything!

Makes: 1 cup

Prep time: 10 minutes

- ½ cup sunflower seed oil
- ½ cup extra-virgin olive oil
- 2 large egg yolks
- 1 tablespoon Dijon mustard
- 1 tablespoon fresh lemon juice
- ½ teaspoon chipotle powder
- 1 teaspoon sea salt

Combine the sunflower seed oil and olive oil in a measuring cup.

In a blender, combine the egg yolks, mustard, lemon juice, chipotle powder, and salt and process for a few seconds to blend. With the machine running on low speed, add the oil only a few drops at a time. Once the mixture starts to thicken, add the remaining oil in a very slow, thin stream.

Transfer the mayonnaise to a nonreactive container. Use right away or cover tightly and refrigerate for up to 4 days. If the mayonnaise gets too thick, whisk in up to 3 tablespoons cold filtered water to thin it.

Nutritional analysis per serving (1 tablespoon): *Calories: 92, Fat: 9.5 g, Saturated Fat: 1.5 g, Cholesterol: 23 mg, Fiber: 0.5 g, Protein: 1.25 g, Carbohydrates: 1 g, Sodium: 150 mg*

GREEN OLIVE TAPENADE

Makes: 1½ cups

Prep time:
15 minutes

Tapenade is a savory spread made from olives, a staple ingredient in the Mediterranean pantry. The big, bold flavors of tapenade pair well with fish, chicken, lamb, and roasted vegetables.

- 1½ cups green olives, pitted
- 3 garlic cloves, roughly chopped
- ¼ cup hemp seeds
- 8 olive oil–packed anchovies, drained
- grated zest of 1 lemon
- juice of ½ lemon
- 1 teaspoon chopped fresh rosemary
- ½ cup fresh parsley leaves, roughly chopped
- ¼ cup extra-virgin olive oil

In a food processor, combine the olives, garlic, hemp seeds, anchovies, lemon zest and juice, rosemary, and parsley and pulse until the olives are roughly chopped, 4 or 5 pulses. With the machine running, add the olive oil in a steady stream and process until a coarse paste forms, about 1 minute. Scrape down the bowl and pulse a few times to ensure that the mixture is well combined.

Transfer the tapenade to a bowl and serve, or store in an airtight container in the refrigerator for up to 1 week.

Nutritional analysis per serving (¼ cup): Calories: 90, Fat: 7 g, Saturated Fat: 0 g, Cholesterol: 0 mg, Fiber: 1 g, Protein: 3 g, Carbohydrates: 13 g, Sodium: 99 mg

Arugula Pesto

Makes: 1½ cups

Prep time:
15 minutes

Sometimes it's nice to shake things up a bit: This pesto recipe swaps the usual sweet basil for peppery arugula. Nutritional yeast adds a cheesy flavor but keeps the recipe dairy-free.

- 2 cups packed baby arugula
- ⅓ cup pine nuts
- 2 garlic cloves
- ½ cup extra-virgin olive oil
- ¼ cup nutritional yeast
- ½ teaspoon sea salt

In a food processor, combine the arugula, pine nuts, and garlic and pulse until the mixture is finely chopped, 4 or 5 pulses. Scrape down the sides of the bowl, then add the olive oil, nutritional yeast, and salt. Process until well incorporated, about 30 seconds.

Use the pesto right away or refrigerate in an airtight container for up to 1 week. For longer storage, freeze the pesto in ice-cube trays until solid, transfer the cubes to a ziplock bag, and store in the freezer for up to 3 months.

Nutritional analysis per serving (¼ cup): *Calories: 293, Fat: 31 g, Saturated Fat: 4 g, Cholesterol: 0 mg, Fiber: 1 g, Protein: 3 g, Carbohydrates: 3 g, Sodium: 151 mg*

Pecan Romesco

Makes: 2 cups

Prep time:
10 minutes

Cook time:
15 minutes

Romesco is a Spanish sauce made with nuts, tomato, garlic, and peppers or chiles. This version uses pecans instead of the traditional almonds. The bold flavors of Romesco pair well with grilled meats, roasted fish, and roasted vegetables.

- 2 tablespoons extra-virgin olive oil
- 1 large red bell pepper
- 3 plum tomatoes, cored and cut in half
- 2 garlic cloves
- ⅓ cup pecans
- 1 dried Thai red chile, stem removed
- 1 (4-inch) sprig rosemary, leaves only, finely chopped
- 1 tablespoon sherry vinegar
- 2 tablespoons chia seeds, ground in a spice grinder
- 1 teaspoon sea salt

Preheat the oven to 375°F.

In a 10-inch cast-iron skillet, warm the olive oil over medium-high heat until shimmering. Add the bell pepper and cook, turning every 2 minutes, until half of its surfaces are browned. Add the tomato halves skin side down to the pan, along with the garlic. Cook, continuing to turn the bell pepper, until the pepper is browned on all sides and the garlic begins to color, about 2 minutes. Add the pecans, dried chile, and rosemary to the pan. Place the pan in the oven and cook until the pepper and tomatoes are quite soft and tender, about 8 minutes. Remove the pan from the oven and allow the contents to cool completely.

Remove and discard the stem and seeds from the bell pepper and add the flesh to a blender along with the tomatoes, garlic, pecans, dried chile, and rosemary. Scrape any juices and browned bits from the pan into the blender and add the vinegar, chia seeds, and salt. Blend on high speed until the mixture is as smooth as it can be, about 45 seconds.

Use the Romesco right away or refrigerate in an airtight container for up to 4 days.

Nutritional analysis per serving (½ cup): *Calories: 178, Fat: 14 g, Saturated Fat: 2 g, Cholesterol: 0 mg, Fiber: 4 g, Protein: 2 g, Carbohydrates: 10 g, Sodium: 636 mg*

CHIMICHURRI

Makes: about
1 cup

Prep time:
10 minutes

Argentina is known for its high-quality beef, and there chimichurri is the accompaniment of choice for grilled steaks. The sauce's fresh, vibrant flavors are perfect with the richness of red meat, but they're great with poultry, too.

- 1 bunch flat-leaf parsley, stems removed
- 2 tablespoons fresh oregano leaves
- 6 garlic cloves
- ½ cup extra-virgin olive oil
- ¼ cup apple cider vinegar
- 1 teaspoon ground cumin
- 1 teaspoon sea salt
- ½ teaspoon freshly ground black pepper

In a food processor, combine all the ingredients and pulse until just slightly chunky, about 8 pulses.

Use the chimichurri right away or refrigerate in an airtight container for up to 2 weeks.

Nutritional analysis per serving (¼ cup): Calories: 372, Fat: 41 g, Saturated Fat: 6 g, Cholesterol: 0 mg, Fiber: 1 g, Protein: 1 g, Carbohydrates: 2 g, Sodium: 604 mg

ROSEMARY VINAIGRETTE

Makes: about
2 cups

Prep time:
10 minutes

Rosemary is a hardy Mediterranean herb that is said to improve memory and is known for its antibacterial properties. Use this robust vinaigrette on salads or fish or as a marinade for tempeh or chicken.

- 1½ cups extra-virgin olive oil
- ¾ cup apple cider vinegar
- 1 tablespoon whole-grain mustard
- 1 large sprig fresh rosemary, leaves only, finely chopped
- 1 garlic clove
- 1 teaspoon sea salt
- ¼ teaspoon freshly ground black pepper

Combine all the ingredients in a blender and blend on high speed until well combined, about 45 seconds.

Use right away or refrigerate in an airtight container for up to 2 weeks. (If refrigerated, bring to room temperature and whisk to recombine before using.)

Nutritional analysis per serving (¼ cup): Calories: 364, Fat: 44 g, Saturated Fat: 8 g, Cholesterol: 0 mg, Fiber: 0 g, Protein: 0 g, Carbohydrates: 0 g, Sodium: 288 mg

Pine Nut Caesar Dressing

Makes: about
1 cup

Prep time:
5 minutes

Sometimes I miss a good Caesar dressing for romaine lettuce and other greens. This cheese-free version using pine nuts and nutritional yeast will fool anyone with its creamy goodness. It is absolutely possible to achieve a rich, supple texture without using dairy.

- ½ cup pine nuts
- 2 garlic cloves
- 2 tablespoons nutritional yeast
- 1 tablespoon Dijon mustard
- 4 olive oil–packed anchovies
- 2 tablespoons fresh lemon juice
- ½ cup extra-virgin olive oil
- ½ teaspoon sea salt

Combine all the ingredients in a blender and blend on high speed until smooth and creamy, about 1 minute.

Use the dressing right away or refrigerate in an airtight container for up to 1 week.

Nutritional analysis per serving (¼ cup): Calories: 427, Fat: 41 g, Saturated Fat: 5 g, Cholesterol: 3 mg, Fiber: 3 g, Protein: 9 g, Carbohydrates: 7 g, Sodium: 522 mg

Southeast Asian–Style Almond Butter Sauce

Use this flavorful, easy-to-make sauce with homemade chicken nuggets, on kelp or zucchini noodles, or as a dip for vegetable crudités.

Makes: about
2 cups

Prep time:
5 minutes

- ¼ cup full-fat coconut milk
- ¾ cup roasted almond butter
- 1 (1-inch) piece ginger, peeled and grated
- 1 garlic clove
- 2 tablespoons wheat-free tamari
- 2 tablespoons fresh lime juice
- 2 tablespoons rice vinegar
- 1 tablespoon fish sauce
- 1 small dried red chile

Combine all the ingredients in a blender and blend on high speed until creamy, about 45 seconds.

Use the sauce right away or transfer to an airtight container and refrigerate for up to 1 week.

Nutritional analysis per serving (2 tablespoons): *Calories: 52, Fat: 3 g, Saturated Fat: 0 g, Cholesterol: 0 mg, Fiber: 1 g, Protein: 2 g, Carbohydrates: 2 g, Sodium: 159 mg*

Smoky Ketchup

PEGAN DIET

Have you ever looked at the ingredients in commercial ketchup? Sugar of some kind is usually near the top of the list. People always tell me they miss ketchup for spreading on a burger or for dipping sweet potato fries. So I had to include a Pegan version in this collection of recipes! Here's a ketchup that's sugar-free and gets a spicy, lightly smoky flavor from chipotle powder.

- ¼ cup tomato paste
- 1 small shallot, thinly sliced
- 2 tablespoons apple cider vinegar
- 2 teaspoons Dijon mustard
- ½ teaspoon chipotle powder
- ½ teaspoon ground allspice
- ⅛ teaspoon ground cloves
- ½ teaspoon sea salt
- 2 dates, pitted

In a small, heavy-bottom saucepan, combine all the ingredients and pour in 1½ cups filtered water. Bring to a simmer over medium heat and cook, stirring occasionally, until the water evaporates and the mixture thickens, 15 to 20 minutes.

Using an immersion blender, puree the mixture in the saucepan until smooth. Alternatively, transfer the mixture to a blender and blend on high speed until smooth.

Use the ketchup right away or refrigerate in an airtight container for up to 1 week.

Nutritional analysis per serving (2 tablespoons): *Calories: 60, Fat: 0 g, Saturated Fat: 0 g, Cholesterol: 0 mg, Fiber: 4 g, Protein: 0 g, Carbohydrates: 16 g, Sodium: 652 mg*

GINGERY BARBECUE SAUCE

Like ketchup, most store-bought barbecue sauces are laden with sugar. Still, I love good barbecue sauce, so here's one that has all the right tangy, sweet, and spicy flavors, but without any added sugar. This sauce pairs well with chicken, but I also enjoy it slathered on roasted cauliflower, grilled portobello mushrooms, tempeh, and tofu.

Makes: 2 cups

Prep time: 15 minutes

Cook time: 1 hour, plus cooling time

- 1 (28-ounce) can whole peeled tomatoes
- 2 tablespoons extra-virgin olive oil
- 1 large yellow onion, finely chopped
- 1 (2-inch) piece ginger, peeled and minced
- 3 garlic cloves, minced
- ½ cup apple cider vinegar
- ½ cup wheat-free tamari
- 1 whole star anise
- 1 teaspoon ground allspice
- ¼ teaspoon sea salt
- ¼ teaspoon freshly ground black pepper

In a food processor, pulse the tomatoes with their juice until coarsely pureed, 3 or 4 pulses.

In a medium heavy-bottom saucepan, warm the olive oil over medium heat until shimmering. Add the onion and cook, stirring occasionally, until softened and translucent, 4 to 5 minutes. Stir in the ginger and garlic and cook until fragrant, about 2 minutes. Pour in the vinegar and allow to reduce by half. Add 1½ cups filtered water and the tamari, star anise, allspice, salt, and pepper and simmer, stirring occasionally, until the sauce has thickened and reduced to 2 cups, about 45 minutes. Allow to cool completely.

Use the sauce right away or refrigerate in an airtight container for up to 5 days.

Nutritional analysis per serving (½ cup): *Calories: 245, Fat: 10 g, Saturated Fat: 0 g, Cholesterol: 0 mg, Fiber: 10 g, Protein: 5 g, Carbohydrates: 45 g, Sodium: 2195 mg*

Classic Tomato Sauce

Makes: 8 cups

Prep time:
5 minutes

Cook time:
8 hours, 20
minutes
(mostly
unattended)

Every home cook needs a good recipe for tomato sauce. Once you see how simple it is to make and how great the results taste, you'll never buy jarred sauce again. I like to make large batches and freeze the sauce by the quart so I have some available at a moment's notice. The trick to a good tomato sauce is to simmer slowly and stir occasionally—with a wooden spoon, of course!

- 2 (28-ounce) cans whole peeled tomatoes
- 2 tablespoons extra-virgin olive oil
- 5 garlic cloves, crushed
- 3 tablespoons tomato paste
- 2 teaspoons dried thyme
- 1 teaspoon dried oregano
- 1 bay leaf
- 2 cups loosely packed basil leaves, torn into small pieces
- 2 teaspoons sea salt
- ½ teaspoon freshly ground black pepper

In a blender, puree the tomatoes with their juice until smooth.

In a large, heavy saucepan, warm the olive oil over medium-high heat until shimmering. Add the garlic and cook, stirring frequently, until golden brown, 2 to 3 minutes. Stir in the tomato paste and cook until slightly darkened in color, about 2 minutes. Carefully pour in the pureed tomatoes, add the thyme, oregano, and bay leaf, and pour in 8 cups filtered water. Bring to a boil, then reduce the heat to medium, cover partially, and simmer, stirring occasionally, until the sauce is quite thick and reduced to 8 cups, about 8 hours.

Add the basil and continue to simmer to allow the flavors to mingle, about 15 minutes. Stir in the salt and pepper. Use the sauce right away, store it in an airtight container in the refrigerator for up to 4 days, or freeze for up to 6 months.

Nutritional analysis per serving (½ cup): *Calories: 148, Fat: 8 g, Saturated Fat: 2 g, Cholesterol: 0 mg, Fiber: 8 g, Protein: 4 g, Carbohydrates: 18 g, Sodium: 952 mg*

GHEE

Ghee, the cooking fat of choice in India, has a wonderfully rich flavor and is very simple to make at home using unsalted, grass-fed butter. Because ghee is pure butterfat and free of milk solids, those with lactose sensitivities usually do fine with ghee. This recipe makes 2 cups, but if you'll be using a lot of ghee in your cooking, you can double the recipe and make a bigger batch—ghee keeps for up to 6 months in the refrigerator.

- 1 pound unsalted, grass-fed butter, cut into cubes

In a small saucepan, warm the butter over medium heat until completely melted and beginning to simmer. Reduce the heat to low and cook without stirring until the butter foams and the foam settles to the bottom of the pan, about 15 minutes. Allow to cool slightly.

Line a fine-mesh sieve with several layers of cheesecloth and set the sieve over a bowl. Pour the ghee into the sieve, then transfer to a glass jar and seal tightly.

Store the ghee at room temperature for up to 30 days or in the refrigerator for up to 6 months.

Nutritional analysis per serving (2 tablespoons): *Calories: 200, Fat: 20 g, Saturated Fat: 14 g, Cholesterol: 60 mg, Fiber: 0 g, Protein: 0 g, Carbohydrates: 0 g, Sodium: 0 mg*

HERBED COMPOUND BUTTER

Makes: 1 pound

Prep time:
15 minutes

Compound butter is a fantastic delivery system for rich flavor and good-quality fat. Use this butter on Spiced Sweet Potato Quick Bread (page 251), or melt it into Pegan Diet–approved cooked vegetables and grains. Slice ¼-inch pats of the chilled butter and place them on fish or chicken before baking, or set them on top of just-cooked steaks and allow the butter to melt onto the meat.

- 1 pound unsalted, grass-fed butter, cut into cubes, room temperature
- ½ cup loosely packed fresh parsley leaves
- 2 tablespoons fresh mint leaves, roughly chopped
- 1 tablespoon fresh rosemary leaves, minced
- 2 sprigs thyme, leaves only, roughly chopped
- 2 teaspoons sea salt
- ¼ teaspoon freshly ground black pepper

In a food processor, pulse the butter cubes to break them up, 4 or 5 pulses. Scrape down the bowl and process until the butter is creamy and smooth, about 45 seconds. Add the herbs, salt, and pepper and process until well combined, about 1 minute.

Cut a 12-inch square of parchment paper and lay it on the counter. Scoop the butter onto the bottom quarter of the parchment and form the butter into a log about 4 inches long, using the parchment paper to help you create a compact log. Wrap the log in the parchment and twist the ends so the package resembles a wrapped candy. Refrigerate until the butter is firm, at least 2 hours or up to 6 days, or freeze for up to 3 months.

Nutritional analysis per serving (2 tablespoons): Calories: 212, Fat: 24 g, Saturated Fat: 16 g, Cholesterol: 60 mg, Fiber: 0 g, Protein: 0 g, Carbohydrates: 2 g, Sodium: 290 mg

MEYER LEMON–CHIVE COMPOUND BUTTER

Makes: 1 pound

Prep time:
15 minutes

The Meyer lemon, a cross between the common orange and the lemon, has a lemon-like flavor, but with less acidity and a touch more sweetness. Use this compound butter on chicken, fresh wild salmon, or halibut. You won't be able to get enough of it!

- 2 garlic cloves
- 1 teaspoon sea salt
- 1 pound unsalted, grass-fed butter, cut into small cubes, room temperature
- grated zest of 4 Meyer lemons
- 2 tablespoons finely chopped fresh chives

Mince the garlic, sprinkle it with the salt, and continue to mince until the garlic forms a paste.

In a stand mixer fitted with the flat-beater attachment, beat the butter until smooth and creamy, 2 to 3 minutes. Alternatively, process the butter in a food processor for 1 minute. Scrape down the sides of the bowl. Add the garlic paste, lemon zest, and chives and mix until well combined.

Cut a 12-inch sheet of parchment paper and lay it on the counter. Scoop the butter onto the bottom quarter of the parchment and form the butter into a log about 5 inches long, using the parchment paper to help you shape a compact log. Wrap the log in the parchment and twist the ends so the package resembles a wrapped candy. Refrigerate until the butter is firm, at least 2 hours or up to 6 days, or freeze for up to 3 months.

Nutritional analysis per serving (2 tablespoons): *Calories: 200, Fat: 22 g, Saturated Fat: 14 g, Cholesterol: 60 mg, Fiber: 0 g, Protein: 0 g, Carbohydrates: 0 g, Sodium: 144 mg*

PICKLED KOHLRABI

Makes: 4 cups

Prep time:
20 minutes,
plus 3 to 4 days
for
fermentation

From sauerkraut to kimchi, naturally pickled, or fermented, vegetables are enjoyed by many cultures around the globe. This simple fermentation utilizes kohlrabi, a vegetable in the same family as cabbage and broccoli. These crunchy pickles go well with just about any meal.

- 2 pounds green or purple kohlrabi
- 2 tablespoons sea salt
- 1 teaspoon ground turmeric

Cut off the top and bottom of the kohlrabi, then peel and quarter the bulbs. In a food processor fitted with the medium shredding disk, shred the kohlrabi. Pack the shreds into a 1-quart, wide-mouth Mason jar.

In a medium bowl or 1-quart measuring cup, combine 4 cups lukewarm filtered water and the salt and stir until the salt has completely dissolved. Stir in the turmeric, then pour the mixture over the kohlrabi, filling the jar to just below the rim.

Cover the jar with a piece of cheesecloth and secure with a rubber band. Let stand at room temperature until the liquid becomes bubbly when the jar is gently agitated, 3 to 4 days.

Serve the pickles right away or remove the cheesecloth, cover the jar with its lid, and refrigerate for up to 1 month.

Nutritional analysis per serving (1 cup): Calories: 108, Fat: 5 g, Saturated Fat: 2 g, Cholesterol: 0 mg, Fiber: 3 g, Protein: 4 g, Carbohydrates: 11 g, Sodium: 3973 mg

FRAGRANT SPICE BLEND

Having an assortment of spice blends at the ready will allow you to season different cuts of meat with big, bold flavors even when you're pressed for time. This particular blend is perfect for lamb yet mild enough for use on chicken. Cardamom seeds are the tiny brown or blackish peppercorn-like flecks found inside the cardamom pod. To get the seeds out, gently crush the pod against a work surface, then use your fingers to crack it open and remove the seeds.

Makes: about ½ cup

Prep time: 5 minutes

Cook time: 5 minutes

- 2 tablespoons coriander seeds
- 4 teaspoons cumin seeds
- 2 teaspoons fennel seeds
- 2 small dried red chiles
- 10 cardamom seeds
- 2 tablespoons sea salt

In a small skillet, combine the coriander seeds, cumin seeds, fennel seeds, chiles, and cardamom seeds. Set the pan over medium-high heat and toast the spices, shaking the pan continuously, until very fragrant, 3 to 4 minutes.

Transfer the spices to a spice grinder and process until finely ground and powdery. (Alternatively, use a mortar and pestle to grind the spices.) Transfer the spice mixture to an airtight container and stir in the salt. Use the spice blend right away or seal the container and store at room temperature for up to 6 months.

Nutritional analysis per serving (2 tablespoons): Calories: 17, Fat: 1 g, Saturated Fat: 0 g, Cholesterol: 0 mg, Fiber: 2 g, Protein: 0 g, Carbohydrates: 3 g, Sodium: 1683 mg

Sofrito

Makes: about
4 cups

Prep time:
10 minutes

Cook time:
35 minutes,
plus cooling
time

Sofrito is the traditional flavor base for many Latin American and Spanish dishes. While sofrito ingredients may differ from region to region, the mixture always contains aromatic vegetables, such as onions, peppers, and garlic, that are cooked slowly to concentrate the flavors and allow them to meld. Use sofrito as a seasoning for meats and roasted veggies or stir some into cooked grains such as rice and quinoa during the Pegan portion of the plan.

- 2 pounds plum tomatoes, cored and roughly chopped
- 2 large red bell peppers, seeded and roughly chopped
- 2 large yellow onions, roughly chopped
- 4 large garlic cloves
- 2 tablespoons paprika
- 1 teaspoon smoked paprika
- 2 tablespoons extra-virgin olive oil or rendered lard

In a large bowl, toss together the tomatoes, bell peppers, onions, and garlic.

Working in two or three batches, in a food processor, pulse the vegetables until finely chopped, 4 or 5 pulses, and transfer to a medium bowl. Stir the paprika and smoked paprika into the chopped vegetables.

In a large saucepan, warm the olive oil over medium-high heat until shimmering. Add the vegetable mixture and cook, stirring occasionally, until thickened and reduced to about 4 cups, 25 to 30 minutes.

Allow the sofrito to cool completely. Transfer to an airtight container and refrigerate for up to 2 weeks or freeze for up to 6 months.

Nutritional analysis per serving (½ cup): *Calories: 85, Fat: 4 g, Saturated Fat: 1 g, Cholesterol: 0 mg, Fiber: 3 g, Protein: 2 g, Carbohydrates: 14 g, Sodium: 14 mg*

16

7-Day *Eat Fat, Get Thin* Meal Plan

I can talk about the importance of cutting out processed sugars and carbohydrates and eating plenty of plant foods and healthy fats, but everyone wants to know: Do I walk the talk? The truth is, I have to. I have about ten jobs, two kids, a dog, a work team, weeks and weeks of travel at a time, and the list goes on and on. In order to keep up with this lifestyle, maintaining excellent health becomes a top priority. Thankfully, I prefer the taste of real food over processed junk, and once you reap the benefits of optimal health, turning back isn't even an option.

My day usually starts with some movement—a bike ride, a run, a yoga class, or a game of basketball with my son. When I have a long day ahead of me or I am planning on being extra active, I like to have a little Bulletproof Coffee (page 67), which keeps me satiated for hours. I also will have a smoothie or make some eggs or another delicious, full-fat breakfast dish. For lunch, I enjoy salad on weekdays, and on the weekends, if I have time, I'll prepare something a little more intricate. For dinner, we go all out. I love to cook with my son and daughter if they are in town. We invite a group of friends over and enjoy great conversation and amazing food.

I've created a 7-Day Meal Plan to show you what a week on the *Eat Fat, Get Thin* diet looks like. This plan does not need to be followed to the letter. You can make extras of one recipe for leftovers, or you can replace recipes with any other meal that fits your fancy in this book. This is just an example of a meal plan that I might put together when I am at home in Massachusetts. For dinner, I always recommend making multiple side dishes, which you can find starting on page 148. Variety is key for me, so this meal plan has a little bit of everything.

	Monday	Tuesday	Wednesday	Thursday	Friday	Saturday	Sunday
Breakfast	Chocolate-Raspberry Smoothie (page 66)	Buttery Broccoli and Spinach with Fried Eggs (page 71)	Minted Green Smoothie with Raspberries (page 63)	Southwestern Tofu Scramble (page 81)	Creamy Strawberry and Greens Smoothie (page 61)	Walnut Pancakes with Blueberries (page 82)	Mushroom and Egg Scramble (page 77)
Lunch	Chicken and Arugula Salad with Roasted Red Pepper Vinaigrette (page 121)	Taco Salad (page 125)	Mediterranean Sardine Salad (page 120)	Za'atar Roasted Chicken (page 216)	Hearty Spinach Salad (page 113) + Rich Onion Soup (page 139)	Turkey Burgers with Peppers and Onions (page 220)	Farmers' Market Salad with Miso Dressing (page 108)
Dinner	"Spaghetti" and Meatballs with Tomato Sauce (page 226)	Seared Scallops with Curried Brussels Sprout Slaw (page 193)	Balsamic Beef Stew (page 235) and Shaved Asparagus and Radicchio Salad (page 111)	Thai Red Curry with Seafood and Vegetables (page 196)	Braised Lamb Shanks with Moroccan Flavors (page 248)	Shrimp with Sweet Potatoes, Kale, and Coconut Milk (page 191)	Pot Roast (page 233)

SHOPPING LIST FOR THE 7-DAY MEAL PLAN

Fruit

8 ripe Hass avocados

1 cup fresh blueberries

3 lemons

3 limes

2 navel oranges

Vegetables

1 bunch asparagus

2 crowns broccoli

1 pound Brussels sprouts

1 red cabbage

4 pounds carrots

1 bunch celery

1 pint cherry tomatoes

2 pounds cremini mushrooms

1 large cucumber

2 (2-inch) pieces ginger

1 pound green beans

1 large green bell pepper

4 large red bell peppers
1 bunch radishes
1 large spaghetti squash
2 large summer squash
2 large sweet potatoes
2 large tomatoes
1 pound turnips

1 large zucchini
5 bulbs garlic
2 small red onions
1 large shallot
15 large yellow onions
2 bunches scallions

Greens, Herbs

13 ounces arugula
32 ounces mixed baby greens
1 bunch lacinato kale
1½ pounds baby spinach
1 head radicchio

1 small bunch fresh rosemary
3 bunches cilantro
1 bunch fresh basil
1 bunch fresh thyme
2 bunches flat-leaf parsley

Meat, Fish, Poultry

3 dozen eggs
2 pounds grass-fed ground beef
1½ pounds beef stew meat
1 (2-pounds) beef bottom round
    roast
8 pounds soup bones
1 (3- to 4-pound) boneless
    chicken breasts

4 chicken legs
4 lamb shanks
1 pound mussels
4 (4.37-ounce) cans sardines in
    water or olive oil
1½ pounds scallops
1½ pounds U16 shrimp
1 pound ground turkey

Nuts, Seeds

2½ cups almonds (for nut milk)
⅛ cup chia seeds
1 cup hazelnuts
¼ cup hemp seeds

¼ cup pine nuts
¼ cup pumpkin seeds
¼ cup raw sunflower seeds
1 cup walnuts

Grocery

2 (13.5-ounce) cans full-fat
    unsweetened coconut milk

2 cups beef stock
1 jar ghee

1 package kombu

1 jar roasted red peppers

1 jar olive oil–marinated sun-dried tomatoes

1 (28-ounce) jar fire-roasted tomatoes

1 (7-ounce) glass jar tomato paste (Bionaturae)

1 bottle tomato puree

1 small jar Dijon mustard

1 small jar whole-grain mustard

2 cups pitted Kalamata olives

1 jar red curry paste

1 box peppermint tea bags

1 bottle red wine vinegar

1 (16-ounce) bottle apple cider vinegar

1 jar wheat-free tamari

1 liter extra-virgin olive oil

1 jar coconut oil

1 liter avocado oil

1 small bottle sherry vinegar

1 small bottle balsamic vinegar

1 small bottle fish sauce

1 small bottle white wine vinegar or champagne vinegar

3 cups (1-pound bag) coconut flour

8 ounces arrowroot powder

8 ounces cacao powder

Spices

1 pound sea salt

1 small jar ground white pepper

1 small jar curry powder

1 jar whole black peppercorns

1 small jar cayenne pepper

2 ounces chipotle powder

2 ounces chili powder

2 ounces ground cinnamon

2 ounces ground coriander seed

2 ounces ground cumin

1 small jar fennel seeds

1 small jar garlic powder

1 small jar red pepper flakes

1 small container saffron threads

1 small jar turmeric

1 small jar dried thyme

1 small jar dried oregano

1 small jar za'atar seasoning

1 jar bay leaves

1 teaspoon vanilla powder

1 (2-ounce) bottle alcohol-free, gluten-free pure vanilla flavoring

1 small container aluminum-free baking powder

1 small container baking soda

Refrigerated Items

1 pound unsalted, grass-fed
   butter
1 block firm (organic, non-
   GMO) tofu

1 jar soy-free miso (South River
   Miso)

Specialty

1 preserved lemon
1 bottle MCT oil

1 bottle organic dry white wine
1 bottle organic red wine

Frozen

ice cubes
1 (10-ounce) pack frozen raspberries
1 (10-ounce) pack frozen strawberries

Acknowledgments

My vision for this cookbook was to prove once and for all that food can taste good and be good for you *and* that we can and should have healthy relationships with our bodies, our kitchens, and the food we eat. Even though the misguided advice to avoid fats and embrace processed carbohydrates we've heard for decades is still being preached by many doctors, scientists, and even the media, the response to *Eat Fat, Get Thin* has proved to me that we are no longer interested in tasteless, low-fat meals and outdated research. Achieving real, lasting results with real food and enjoying the process is what this book is all about.

This vision would not be possible without you—without anyone who believes that they can transform their health with the power of food. In order to change the health of the world, we need to start with ourselves, so thank *you* for investing in this journey with me.

To help create these deeply satisfying and delectable meals, I knew that I had to find a chef who shared my affection for healthy fats and real, whole foods. My friend Chef Frank Giglio is the first person I thought of. I have never tasted a recipe of his that I didn't love. He has spent a great deal of time creating mouthwatering meals that are designed for maximum nutrition.

For bringing these recipes to life, I'd like to thank our photographer, Leela Cyd, and food stylist, Ayda Robana, as well as their teams for capturing all of these beautiful meals. I want to give special thanks to Kaya Purohit, who worked tirelessly on every page, making this book great. I could not do half of what I do without you. Thank you. And, of course,

Dhru Purohit, my business partner, who steers the ship, leads the troops, and makes it all happen!

Of course, none of this would be possible without the people who have kept this book organized—my team at Little, Brown, especially my editor, Tracy Behar, and Jean Garnett. I'd also like to thank my agent, Richard Pine, as well as the Hyman Digital team and my team at The UltraWellness Center and the Cleveland Clinic Center for Functional Medicine for their tremendous amount of support and for helping me spread the message that food *is* medicine.

Resources

FURTHER READING AND RESOURCES FROM MARK HYMAN, MD

Mark Hyman's Websites
www.drhyman.com
www.eatfatgetthin.com
www.10daydetox.com
www.bloodsugarsolution.com

The UltraWellness Center
55 Pittsfield Road, Suite 9
Lenox Commons
Lenox, MA 01240
(413) 637-9991
www.ultrawellnesscenter.com

Cleveland Clinic Center for Functional Medicine
9500 Euclid Avenue
Cleveland, OH 44195
(216) 445-6900 or toll-free at (844) 833-0126

I am the founder and director of The UltraWellness Center and the director of the Cleveland Clinic Center for Functional Medicine. Both of these teams consist of trained and experienced Functional Medicine physicians, nutritionists, nurses, and health coaches who can guide you through diet and lifestyle changes, as well as specialized testing, nutritional supplementation, and medications.

Books and Programs

Eat Fat, Get Thin (book and public television special)

The Blood Sugar Solution 10-Day Detox Diet (book and public television special)

The Blood Sugar Solution 10-Day Detox Diet Cookbook (book)

The Blood Sugar Solution (book and public television special)

The Blood Sugar Solution Cookbook (book)

The UltraMind Solution (book and public television special)

Six Weeks to an UltraMind (audio/DVD program)

The Daniel Plan (book)

The Daniel Plan Cookbook (book)

UltraCalm (audio program)

UltraMetabolism (book and public television special)

The UltraMetabolism Cookbook (book)

The UltraSimple Diet (book)

The UltraThyroid Solution (e-book)

UltraPrevention (book)

The Five Forces of Wellness (audio program)

The Detox Box (audio/DVD program)

Nutrigenomics (audio program)

General References and Resources

Eat Fat, Get Thin Resources

For quizzes, supplement protocol, tracking tools, and all other recommendations, head to www.eatfatgetthin.com/resources, where you will find everything you need.

Environmental Working Group

www.ewg.org

The Environmental Working Group empowers people to live healthier lives in a healthier environment. Use this site to download the guide "Good Food on a Tight Budget" and the "Clean Fifteen/ Dirty Dozen" produce list.

Thrive Market

For wholesome foods for wholesale prices plus my favorite snacks, visit www.thrivemarket.com/efgt. They have all your kitchen staples in one place.

General Index

Recipe Index

About the Author

Mark Hyman, MD, believes that we all deserve a life of vitality—and that we have the potential to create it for ourselves. That's why he is dedicated to tackling the root causes of chronic disease by harnessing the power of Functional Medicine to transform health care. Dr. Hyman and his team work every day to empower people, organizations, and communities to heal their bodies and minds and to improve our social and economic resilience.

Dr. Hyman is a practicing family physician, a ten-time *New York Times* bestselling author, and an internationally recognized leader, speaker, educator, and advocate in his field. He is the Pritzker Foundation Chair in Functional Medicine at Cleveland Clinic and the director of the Cleveland Clinic Center for Functional Medicine. He is also the founder and director of The UltraWellness Center, chairman of the board of the Institute for Functional Medicine, a medical editor of *The Huffington Post,* and he has been a regular medical contributor on many television shows and networks, including *CBS This Morning, Today, Good Morning America,* CNN, *The View, Katie,* and *The Dr. Oz Show.*

Dr. Hyman works with individuals and organizations, as well as policy makers and influencers. He has testified before both the White House Commission on Complementary and Alternative Medicine and the Senate Working Group on Health Care Reform on Functional Medicine. He has consulted with the surgeon general on diabetes prevention, and participated in the 2009 White House Forum on Prevention and Wellness. Senator Tom Harkin of Iowa nominated Dr. Hyman for the

President's Advisory Group on Prevention, Health Promotion, and Integrative and Public Health. In addition, Dr. Hyman has worked with President Bill Clinton, presenting at the Clinton Foundation's Health Matters, Achieving Wellness in Every Generation conference, and the Clinton Global Initiative, as well as with the World Economic Forum on global health issues. He is the winner of the Linus Pauling Award and the Nantucket Project Award, was inducted into the Books for a Better Life Hall of Fame, and received the Christian Book of the Year Award for *The Daniel Plan*.

Dr. Hyman also works with fellow leaders in his field to help people and communities thrive — with Rick Warren, Dr. Mehmet Oz, and Dr. Daniel Amen, he created The Daniel Plan, a faith-based initiative that helped the Saddleback Church collectively lose 250,000 pounds. He is an advisor and guest cohost on *The Dr. Oz Show* and is on the board of Dr. Oz's HealthCorps, which tackles the obesity epidemic by educating American students about nutrition. With Dr. Dean Ornish and Dr. Michael Roizen, Dr. Hyman crafted and helped introduce the Take Back Your Health Act of 2009 to the United States Senate to provide for reimbursement of lifestyle treatment of chronic disease. And with Tim Ryan in 2015, he helped introduce the ENRICH Act into Congress to fund nutrition in medical education. Dr. Hyman plays a substantial role in a major film produced by Laurie David and Katie Couric, released in 2014, called *Fed Up,* which addresses childhood obesity. Please join him in helping us all take back our health at drhyman.com, and follow him on Twitter (@markhymanmd), Facebook (facebook.com/drmarkhyman), and Instagram (@markhymanmd).